Pharmacokinetics

Pharmacokinetics

S. B. Hladky

Manchester University Press
Manchester and New York
Distributed exclusively in the USA and Canada by St. Martin's Press

Published by Manchester University Press
Oxford Road, Manchester M13 9PL, UK
and Room 400, 175 Fifth Avenue,
New York, NY 10010, USA

Distributed exclusively in the USA and Canada by
St. Martin's Press, Inc.
175 Fifth Avenue, New York, NY 10010, USA

British Library cataloguing in publication data
Hladky, S. B.
    Pharmacokinetics
    1. Pharmacokinetics
    I. Title
    615.7

Library of Congress cataloging in publication data
Hladky, S. B.
    Pharmacokinetics / S. B. Hladky
        p. cm.
    Includes index.
    ISBN 0-7190-3411-6 (cloth), -- ISBN 0-7190-3412-4 (paper)
    1. Pharmacokinetics.   I. Title
    [DNLM 1. Drug Therapy. 2. Pharmacokinetics.   QV 38 H677p]
    RM301.5.H53   1990
    615'.7--dc20
    DNLM/DLC
    for Library of Congress   90-6286

ISBN 0 7190 3411 6 hardback
ISBN 0 7190 3412 4 paperback

Printed in Great Britain
by Biddles Ltd, Guildford and King's Lynn

CONTENTS

PART II THE TIME COURSE OF DRUG CONCENTRATIONS

PREFACE

The pharmacokinetic properties of individual drugs are described, of necessity, in every reference book on drug therapy. This short introduction lays the foundations for understanding and using these descriptions. Most importantly it explains the essential concepts of the subject and discusses the physiological and biochemical processes that govern drug and metabolite concentrations within the body. It also defines area under the curve and the pharmacokinetic constants, illustrates how they are used, and outlines the methods for calculating their values.

When I started teaching pharmacokinetics I expected to find textbook chapters and monographs that would both explain the processes occurring in the body and introduce the simpler calculations. However, while I found excellent texts for more advanced courses, there was none that I could recommend to accompany a course of five or six lectures. This book is intended to provide a brief but sound introduction in an inexpensive format. The core concepts and their application to anaesthetics are presented in Chapters 1 to 12. Additional topics which some may wish to include are covered in Supplements S1 to S5. A Glossary of the symbols and subscripts used in the text is provided followed by a section of Exercises and Answers.

As an aid to revision the main points throughout the book are emphasized by bold print.

The name, pharmacokinetics, frequently conjures up an image of detailed, multi-compartment, mathematical models being used to interpret changes in the plasma concentration of drugs. These models continue to have their place. However, in clinical practice average concentrations are far more important than the details of the variations. Reflecting this priority the account given here emphasizes average concentrations and describes the changes in the simplest adequate terms. Curve fitting and models with two or more compartments are introduced briefly in the last two supplements but these topics may be omitted completely from an introductory course.

While the presentation of material in this book is my own and the mistakes are solely my responsibility, the concepts and data have, of course, been taken from others. In the interest of brevity, specific citations are not given except where I have taken experimental values from a source other than Appendix II in Goodman & Gilman.

I owe thanks for helpful advice and criticism to many students and staff members of the Pharmacology Department, but especially to B.A. Callingham, D.R. Ferguson and C.R. Hiley. I would also like to thank L. Aarons, G.R. Park, K. Parks, P.A. Routledge, T. Shepherd, and P. Woods for very generously reading and criticizing versions of the manuscript and K.R. Harrap, P.A. Routledge, K. Smith and P. Workman for providing material from which I've constructed exercises.

I would greatly appreciate it if anyone who finds mistakes or has suggestions for improvements would write and tell me.

FURTHER READING

WHERE TO START

Gibaldi, M. (1984), *Biopharmaceutics and Clinical Pharmacokinetics, 3rd ed.*, Lea & Febiger, Philadelphia. 330pp.

Gibson, G.G. & Skett, P. (1986), *Introduction to Drug Metabolism.* Chapman and Hall, London. 293pp.

Gilman, A.G., Goodman, L.S., Rall, T.W. & Murad, F. (1985), *Goodman and Gilman's The Pharmacological Basis of Therapeutics, 7th ed.* Macmillan, N.Y. 1839pp.

Greenblatt, D.J. & Shader, R.I. (1985), *Pharmacokinetics in Clinical Practice*, Saunders, Philadelphia. 126pp. A qualitative, introductory account. Benzodiazepines.

Rowland, M. & Tozer, T.N. (1989), *Clinical Pharmacokinetics: Concepts and Applications, 2nd ed.*, Lea & Febiger, Philadelphia. 541pp.

GENERAL REFERENCES

Benet, L.Z., Massoud, N. & Gambertoglio, J.G. (1984), *Pharmacokinetic Basis for Drug Treatment*, Raven Press, N.Y. 466pp.

Bowman, W.C. & Rand ,M.J. (1980), *Textbook of Pharmacology*, 2nd ed., Blackwell, Oxford. ca.1900pp. Chapters 26 & 40: many helpful lists and tables.

Curry, S. (1980), *Drug Disposition and Pharmacokinetics, 3rd ed.*, Blackwell, Oxford. 330pp.

Gibaldi, M. & Perrier, D. (1982), *Pharmacokinetics, 2nd ed.* Marcel Dekker, N.Y. 494pp. An advanced mathematical treatment.

Gibaldi, M. & Prescott, L. (1983), *Handbook of Clinical Pharmacokinetics*, ADIS Health Science Press, N.Y. 1184pp.

Gillies, H.C., Rogers, H.J., Spector, R.G. & Trounce, J.R. (1986), *A Textbook of Clinical Pharmacology, 2nd ed.*, Hodder and Stoughton, London. 920pp.

Goldstein, A., Aronow, L. & Kalman, S.M. (1974), *Principles of Drug Action: The Basis of Pharmacology, 2nd ed.*, Wiley, N.Y. 854pp. Classic account of the principles. Anaesthetics.

Grahame-Smith, D.G. & Aronson, J.K. (1987), *Oxford Textbook of Clinical Pharmacology and Drug Therapy*, Oxford University Press, Oxford. 843pp.

Melmon, K.L. & Morrelli, H.F. (1978), *Clinical Pharmacology. Basic Principles in Therapeutics, 2nd ed.*, Macmillan, N.Y. 1146pp.

Prys-Roberts, C. & Hug, C.C.Jr. (1984), *Pharmacokinetics of Anaesthesia*, Blackwell Scientific Publications, Oxford. 358pp.

Saunders, L., Ingram, D. & Jackson, S.H.D. (1989), *Human Drug Kinetics. A Course of Simulated Experiments*, IRL Press, Oxford. 261pp. A computer disk is included. The use of simulation is particularly valuable as an aid to understanding non-linear kinetics.

1 INTRODUCTION

Drugs are prescribed and taken to produce particular results. **Pharmacokinetics describes the processes that determine the concentrations of a drug and its metabolites within the body.** How the effects that are produced depend on these concentrations is considered in pharmacodynamics. While it can be artificial this division of the dose-effect relation into dose-concentration and concentration-effect components is often useful and adequate. It is also the starting point for all other descriptions.

For any drug the concentrations near its sites of action are the most important. Nevertheless plasma concentrations play a central role in pharmacokinetics for both technical and fundamental reasons. In practice plasma concentrations are usually the easiest to measure. But in addition they must be included in any description because, as part of the blood, the plasma delivers substances to and removes them from all the tissues of the body. As a rule, changes in a drug's plasma concentration lead to changes in both the concentration at its site of action and the effects it produces. However, this rule has many exceptions. Reasons include effects produced by metabolites rather than the drug itself (see Section 5.5); slow penetration of the drug to the site of action (see Section S1.2); and irreversible or hit-and-run effects such as the bactericidal action of some antibiotics. These and other complications require that reference books discuss separately the properties of each therapeutic agent. Nevertheless **all pharmacokinetic descriptions, with or without complications, rely on a common set of basic principles.**

The ideal time course of the plasma concentration for many drugs looks something like the solid curve in Fig.1.1. To achieve a sustained therapeutic effect the concentration must be raised to an effective level and either maintained at or repeatedly brought back to this level over a period of time. To minimize toxicity the concentration must not be too high and, when treatment is complete, it should fall rapidly. Only rarely can a single dose produce adequate concentrations.

Drugs are eliminated from the body either by their excretion or by their conversion into other substances by metabolism. Because elimination occurs at all times, not just at the end of treatment, when a single dose is given the plasma concentration doesn't hover at a constant level. It goes up and then comes back

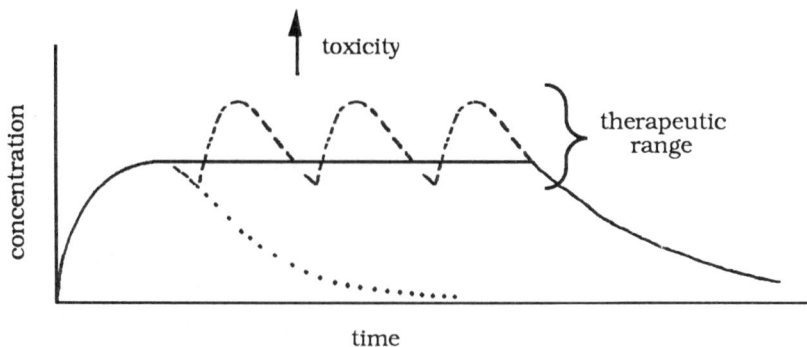

Figure 1.1 Comparison of an "ideal" time course for plasma concentration (——) with the concentrations resulting from a single dose (....) alone or with top-up doses (- - -).

down. To keep the concentration above a minimum level, top-up doses must be given at regular intervals to replace the portion that has been eliminated. After each of these additional doses, the concentration again goes up to a peak and falls, so that a more realistic concentration time curve looks a bit like the teeth of a saw.

These simple considerations illustrate several important pharmacokinetic questions.

(1)   What concentrations are required for the desired effect?

(2)   At what maintenance rate must the drug reach the general circulation to maintain a desired concentration?

(3)   To what extent is an administered dose actually absorbed into the body?

(4)   How much drug must be accumulated within the body to reach and sustain a desired concentration?

(5)   How long after one dose until the next one must be given? In other words how rapidly does the drug concentration fall after each dose?

The experimental answers to questions like these are collected together in the standard references of pharmacology. For instance data for more than 150 drugs are tabulated in Appendix 2 of Goodman & Gilman. This information is reported in terms of effective and toxic plasma concentrations (an attempt to "answer" question 1) and a standard set of pharmacokinetic constants which includes the clearance (question 2), the availability (question 3), the steady-state volume of distribution (question 4), and the half-life (question 5). For many drugs these constants provide all the information that is needed to calculate doses that will usually keep the plasma concentration and the effects produced within the therapeutic range. The calculations are only approximate, but there is little point in making them more accurate because both the concentrations required and those actually produced differ from one occasion to another.

Changes in how a person's body handles a drug can alter the effects of the drug on the body. The changes of greatest clinical importance are those that alter the concentrations averaged over the period of treatment. For this reason the most important sections of this book are this Introduction, Chapters 2 to 5 on elimination, and Chapter 6 on absorption. It may seem back to front to consider how drugs are eliminated before discussing how they are administered. However, elimination can be studied while absorption is not occurring, but absorption is always accompanied by elimination.

1.1 CONCENTRATIONS

Before any of the pharmacokinetic constants can be defined or used it is first necessary to be careful about what is meant by "the concentration of a drug".

1.1.1 Free and total concentrations

After a substance has been dissolved in a body fluid, the individual molecules may be found free in solution or bound to something else like soluble proteins, connective tissue, or cell membranes. Some, rarely more than a small proportion, may interact with specific receptors. For almost all drugs, binding occurs rapidly and, providing the drug isn't then covalently bonded or metabolized, so does dissociation. Thus in most instances, if the concentration of free drug changes, that of bound drug changes as well. In other words in each small region of the body, e.g. just outside a cell or in a cell's cytoplasm, the free and bound forms remain at equilibrium with each other. The total concentration is the sum of the concentrations of the free and bound forms.

In plasma the relative proportions free and bound are stated as either the percentage of the drug in plasma that is bound,

$$b = 100\frac{C^{bound}}{C}$$

or as the fraction of the drug in plasma that is free,

$$f = \frac{C^{free}}{C} = 1 - \frac{b}{100}$$

where C^{free} is the plasma concentration of free drug, C^{bound} that of bound drug, and $C = C^{free} + C^{bound}$ is the total plasma concentration.

Reversible binding to a site or receptor is proportional to the free rather than the total concentration near the site. For the same free concentration, the binding is not affected by changes in the amount bound to other, independent sites. Thus unless a drug's actions are irreversible **the free rather than the total concentration at the site of action determines the effects that can be produced.** Furthermore if the free concentration in the plasma reaching a tissue exceeds that which would be at equilibrium with the tissue, drug will tend to enter the tissue and vice versa. **Free concentrations govern the movements of the drug between plasma and the tissues.** The amount present in a small region or carried in a small volume of plasma is, however, proportional to the total concentration.

Free concentrations are undoubtedly of primary importance in the mechanisms of drug action and in the processes described by pharmacokinetics. (In the language of the physical chemist free concentrations rather than total concentrations are closely related to activities and chemical potentials.) **Nevertheless the total rather than the free plasma concentration is used in most of the equations because even now total concentrations are usually much simpler to measure.** The consequences of plasma protein binding are considered in Section S2.

1.1.2   Effective and toxic concentrations

For most drugs the (minimum) effective concentration is defined as the smallest maintained total plasma concentration that will sustain the desired response. For other drugs, with an effect that outlasts the plasma concentration, e.g. bactericidal antibiotics, the effective concentration is a concentration that must be exceeded at regular intervals.

Toxic concentrations are those that will produce adverse or unwanted effects if they persist for too long.

1.1.3   Plasma concentration measurements in clinical practice

Clinical response is the correct measure of successful administration of a drug. Thus whenever the response is easily observed, plasma concentrations are measured "only" as a means to understand the many processes that intervene between dose and effects. However, for drugs like lithium, theophylline, cyclosporine, methotrexate, aminoglycosides (e.g. gentamicin), cardiac glycosides (e.g. digoxin), and anticonvulsants (e.g. phenytoin) at least some of the effects develop slowly and toxicity is difficult to avoid. For these a more immediate guide to dosing is highly desirable. Comparison of measured plasma concentrations with a target range can provide this guide.

For a target concentration strategy to be worthwhile a number of conditions must be satisfied:

(1)   the clinical response must be difficult to measure in the short term;

(2)   the desired range of concentrations must be known, i.e. it must not vary greatly between individuals;

(3)   the desired range must be sufficiently narrow to make an accurate plasma concentration important;

(4)   the dose-concentration relation must be variable between patients;

(5)   it must be possible to measure the plasma concentration with sufficient sensitivity and specificity and the results of these measurements must be available quickly enough after a blood sample is drawn to allow subsequent doses to be adjusted.

Plasma concentration measurements are also used to investigate unexpected results of standard doses. If the concentrations are as expected the variation usually reflects an unusual sensitivity to the drug. If not, the difficulty may lie in the way the individual absorbs or eliminates the drug. Alternatively it may be that the patient didn't take the drug as prescribed.

PART I
ABSORPTION, ELIMINATION, AVERAGE CONCENTRATIONS AND THE STEADY STATE

2 ELIMINATION AND CLEARANCE

A substance has been eliminated from the body when it has been excreted or chemically changed into something else. The rate of elimination is the sum of the rates of these processes. The clearance of a substance is defined as the ratio

$$CL = \frac{\text{rate of elimination}}{\text{arterial plasma concentration}}$$

While there are important exceptions, for most drugs in clinical use, whenever the plasma concentration changes, the rate of elimination changes in parallel. Following a dose of any of these drugs the plasma concentration and the rate of elimination both vary with time but their ratio, the clearance, remains constant. Because it is constant, the clearance is a particularly economical description of elimination. The processes that determine its value are discussed in Section 2.5 and Chapters 3 to 5.

For an elimination rate in $mmol\,min^{-1}$ and a concentration in $mmol\,ml^{-1}$, the clearance is in $ml\,min^{-1}$, i.e. it has the same units as a flow of fluid. Values usually fall within the range of $1\,ml\,min^{-1}$ to $1000\,ml\,min^{-1}$. Because clearances tend to increase with body size, they are often stated either per unit body weight or per unit body surface area. Weight is commonly used because it is easy to measure, but surface area is preferred whenever there is a wide range of body sizes, e.g. in paediatrics, in veterinary practice, or in the extrapolation of results from animals to man. The basis of the proportionality between clearance and surface area is presumably that renal and hepatic function reflect a metabolic rate which varies with heat loss and area rather than with weight. A typical clearance of $100\,ml\,min^{-1}$ could be written for the standard $70\,kg$ man with $1.7\,m^2$ surface area as either $1.4\,ml\,min^{-1}\,kg^{-1}$ or $59\,ml\,min^{-1}\,m^{-2}$.

The name "clearance" arises because the clearance equals the maximum flow of arterial blood plasma that could be completely cleared of the substance by eliminating it at a rate, $CL \cdot C$. Put another way, if all the drug elimination were occurring at a single site, the clearance would be the smallest flow of arterial blood plasma that could supply the drug to that site.

2.1   PLASMA CONCENTRATION IN THE STEADY STATE

Drug concentrations in the body have reached a steady state when they remain constant or undergo a regular repeated variation. In the steady state, the average amount of drug in the body is constant and therefore the average rate at which the drug enters the body (see Section 6.4) must be equal to the average rate at which it is being eliminated. When it is constant, **the clearance together with the average rate of absorption, $R_{av,in}$, provide all the information that is needed to calculate the average steady-state concentration in plasma, $C_{av,ss}$,** i.e. the relation

average rate of absorption = average rate of elimination

can be rewritten as

$$R_{av,in} = CL \cdot C_{av,ss}$$

or

$$C_{av,ss} = \frac{R_{av,in}}{CL}$$

For example in a young healthy adult lithium is eliminated by renal excretion with $CL = 25\,ml\,min^{-1} = 1.5\,litre\,hr^{-1}$. If 20 mg is absorbed each 12 hr, the average rate of absorption is $20\,mg/12\,hr = 1.7\,mg\,hr^{-1}$ and the average concentration is $1.7\,mg\,hr^{-1}/1.5\,litre\,hr^{-1} = 1.1\,mg\,litre^{-1}$. In a patient with renal failure and $CL = 10\,ml\,min^{-1}$ the average concentration would be 2.5 times larger, i.e. $2.8\,mg\,litre^{-1}$. **If a drug can be eliminated more rapidly at each concentration, i.e. if the clearance is larger, then the average steady-state concentration will be smaller.**

2.2   AREA UNDER THE CURVE

Larger clearances also mean lower concentrations following a single dose. For drugs with constant clearance this statement can be made quantitative by introducing the concept of area under the curve, AUC (see Fig. 2.1).

The amount absorbed from a single dose must equal the total amount eventually eliminated. This total can be calculated as the sum of the amounts eliminated in many short intervals. During any one of these intervals (see Fig. 2.1a), the rate of elimination is equal to the clearance, CL, times the plasma concentration at that time, C. The amount eliminated is the product of the rate and the length of the interval, Δt, i.e. the amount equals $CL \cdot \Delta t$. The product $C \cdot \Delta t$ can be shown on the graph as the area of a rectangle of width Δt and height C. Thus the amount eliminated in the interval is the clearance times this area. **Provided the clearance is constant,** the sum of the amounts eliminated in all the intervals is the clearance times the sum of all the areas, i.e.

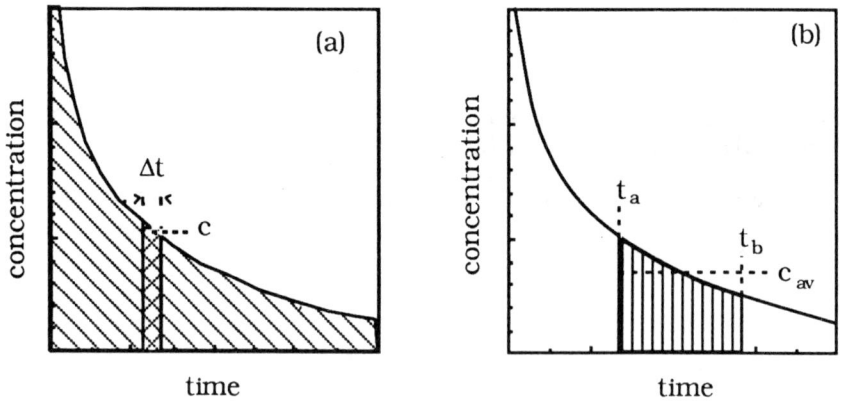

Figure 2.1 Area under the curve and average concentration. The plasma concentration is plotted versus time **on linear scales.** In (a) the product of the length of a short interval of time, Δt, and the concentration during the interval, C, is shown as the cross hatched area. The amount eliminated in this short interval is the clearance times this area. The entire area under the curve, both that shown hatched and the portion not shown for longer times, is called the AUC. It can be calculated by dividing the area into many rectangles like the one shown and adding their areas. If the clearance is constant, the total amount eliminated is equal to $CL \cdot AUC$. In part (b) the average or mean concentration during the interval from t_a to t_b is calculated from the definition of "mean" by dividing the interval into many equal subintervals, adding the concentrations at the midpoints, and dividing this sum by the number of intervals. On the graph the average concentration is the height of a rectangle whose width is $t_b - t_a$ and whose area is equal to the area under the curve between t_a and t_b, i.e.

$$C_{av} \cdot (t_b - t_a) = AUC_{t_a}^{t_b}$$

For curves like that shown, the average concentration for a short interval is close to half-way between the concentrations at the ends of the interval, but for long intervals the average is much smaller than the midpoint.

absorbed dose = amount eventually eliminated = CL · AUC

where AUC is the area under the curve from zero to infinity.

2.3   THE EXPERIMENTAL DETERMINATION OF THE CLEARANCE

Most experimental measurements of the clearance are based on the relation between dose, clearance and total area under the curve,

$$CL = \frac{D}{AUC}$$

The dose may be given as a single rapid injection, called a bolus dose, or preferably as a short infusion (see Fig. 2.2). The plasma concentrations must be measured from the moment drug first enters the body until the amount remaining is negligible. **The simplest correct method for calculating the AUC is to plot the data on ordinary linear graph paper and count all the squares below the curve. The area is then the product of the number of squares and the area of each.** More practical methods for calculating the area are in effect faster ways of counting by taking the squares in groups. Frequently the most convenient method is to describe the curve as a series of straight lines and then calculate the areas of the resulting trapezoids (see Fig. 2.2). Methods for calculating the AUC from initial concentrations and half-lives after an i.v. bolus dose are considered in Section 8.6 and Supplement 4.

The clearance can be calculated as D/AUC only if the AUC is proportional to the dose. If not, elimination is non-linear (see below), the clearance is not a constant, and its value must be measured at each concentration of interest. To make this measurement, the drug is infused at a constant rate, R_0, until the concentration reaches its final value, C_{ss}, and the clearance is calculated as $CL = R_0/C_{ss}$.

2.4   LINEAR VERSUS NON-LINEAR DRUG ELIMINATION

When the rate of elimination is proportional to the plasma concentration, elimination is said to be first order or linear and the clearance is a constant. Doubling the amount of drug given per unit time then doubles the average plasma concentration. This

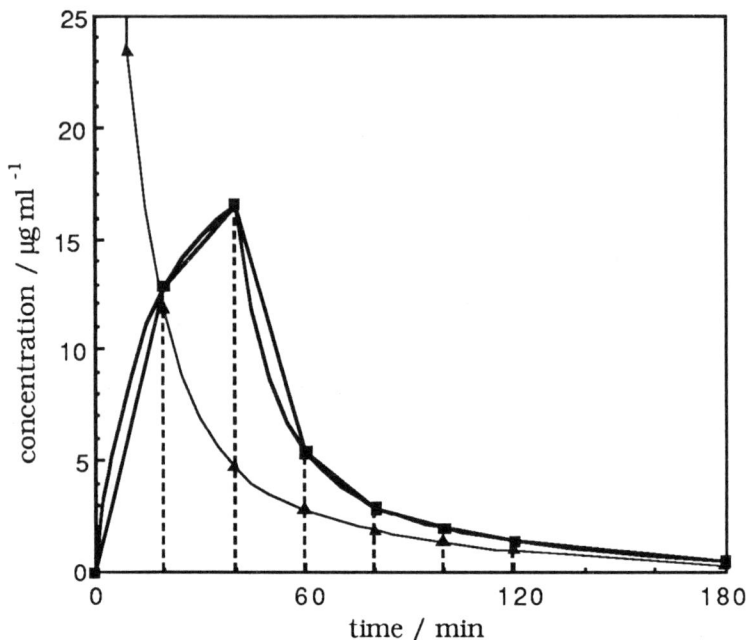

Figure 2.2 Calculation of the AUC after a dose of 500mg of penicillin G administered as an intravenous infusion lasting 60min (the curve with superimposed line segments) or as a single bolus dose (light curve). The AUC's for the two curves are equal, but that for the infusion is much easier to calculate numerically. For this data the AUC is approximately equal to the sum of the area of the triangle and trapezoids that are indicated. The area of the triangle is

$$\frac{1}{2} \cdot base \cdot height = \frac{1}{2} \cdot 20min \cdot C_{20}$$

while that for the trapezoid from 40min to 60min is

$$\frac{1}{2} \cdot base \cdot (sum \ of \ heights) = \frac{1}{2} \cdot 20min \cdot (C_{40} + C_{60})$$

Thus

$$AUC = 20 \ min \left[\frac{1}{2} C_{20} + \frac{1}{2} (C_{20} + C_{40}) + \frac{1}{2} (C_{40} + C_{60}) + \frac{1}{2} (C_{60} + C_{80}) \right.$$
$$\left. + \frac{1}{2} (C_{80} + C_{100}) + \frac{1}{2} (C_{100} + C_{120}) \right] + 60min \cdot \frac{1}{2} (C_{120} + C_{180})$$

$$= 20 \ (6.5 + 14.7 + 10.9 + 4.2 + 2.5 + 1.7) + 60 \ (0.85)$$
$$= 861 \ \mu g \ min \ ml^{-1}.$$

The portion of the AUC in the tail beyond 180 min is missed by this calculation. It can be estimated as $C(180)/\lambda_z$ where λ_z is the terminal phase rate constant described in Chapter 8. Data for practice calculations are given in the Exercises.

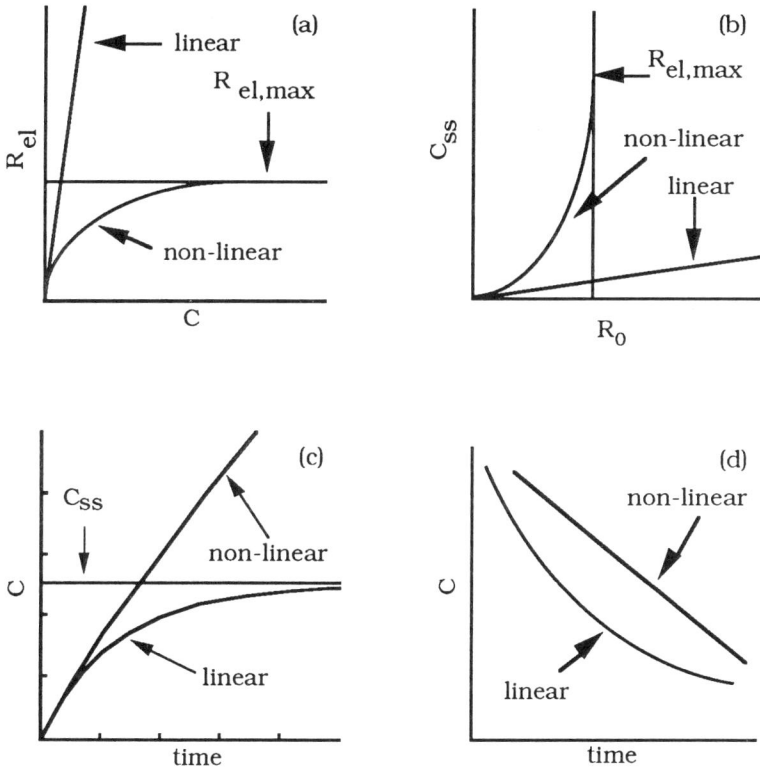

Figure 2.3 A comparison of the consequences of linear elimination, i.e. elimination proportional to plasma concentration, with the consequences of non-linear elimination that cannot exceed a maximum rate, $R_{el,max}$. The curves are drawn assuming that the rates of elimination are the same at low concentrations. (a) Elimination rate versus concentration. (b) Steady-state concentration versus constant infusion rate. (c) Concentration versus time following the start of a constant infusion at rate, $R_0 = 2 R_{el,max}$. (d) Concentration versus time after a large bolus dose. In a) for linear elimination the gradient of the line is the clearance. For non-linear elimination the clearance is the gradient of the chord which decreases as the concentration increases. Because in the steady-state $R_0 = R_{el}$, (b) is just (a) with the horizontal and vertical axes interchanged. In (c) when the elimination is linear, the concentration produced by an infusion increases to a constant, steady-state value, C_{ss}. By contrast when the rate of elimination has a maximum value, infusion at a rate greater than this maximum leads to a continual increase in concentration. For infusion rates below the maximum rate, a steady-state concentration is reached but the variation of this level with the infusion rate is non-linear, see (b). After a large dose, see (d), non-linear, constant rate elimination leads to a linear fall in concentration with time, while for linear elimination, the rate of fall decreases as the concentration decreases and the concentration falls non-linearly with time (see Chapter 8).

simple relation does not apply to all drugs. If elimination occurs primarily by metabolism, and the rate of metabolism is saturable, the results can be quite different (see Fig. 2.3).

An important example, close to the experience of many, is ethanol. Ethanol is eliminated by metabolism. The rate-limiting enzyme, alcohol dehydrogenase saturates at levels corresponding to very mild intoxication. Above these levels the rate of elimination is almost constant. **A steady input of a drug above its maximum rate of elimination leads not to a steady-state plasma level but rather to a relentless increase in the plasma concentration.** Of course with ethanol the concentration never reaches infinity, because consumption stops, voluntarily or otherwise. Afterwards the concentration falls at a constant rate corresponding to the maximum rate of elimination until the metabolic mechanism is no longer saturated. For each additional 20g consumed (about an English pint of beer), intoxication lasts for roughly three more hours. Ethanol is an example of a drug for which the rate of elimination does not vary linearly with the plasma concentration. Non-linear elimination is compared with linear elimination in Fig. 2.3.

Non-linear drug elimination is of critical importance in the clinical use of the anticonvulsant phenytoin. Phenytoin is eliminated by metabolism to an inactive product. The rate of this metabolism has been found experimentally to be described empirically (and approximately) by

$$\text{rate of metabolism} = \frac{7.5\,\text{mg kg}^{-1}\text{day}^{-1} \cdot C}{C + 5.7\,\mu\text{g ml}^{-1}}$$

The rate is linear for low concentrations and approaches a maximum value for high concentrations. Using this relation, the lower end of the therapeutic range of plasma concentrations, about $10\,\mu\text{g ml}^{-1}$, can be maintained with average rates of absorption and elimination somewhere near $7.5 \cdot 10/(10 + 5.7) = 4.8\,\text{mg kg}^{-1}\text{day}^{-1}$. The balance, however, is precarious. Thus in a patient whose maximum rate of elimination is half normal (which isn't unusual), the same average rate of absorption would lead to a concentration that increased further after every dose effectively without limit. Toxic and eventually fatal effects would then be inevitable unless the dose rate, that is the rate of administration, were reduced. Phenytoin dosage must be adjusted individually for each patient (see Section E.2.5).

2.5 ROUTES OF ELIMINATION AND THE ADDITIVITY OF CLEARANCES

Most drugs can be eliminated by more than one route (see Fig. 2.4) and a partial clearance can be defined for each. For example, the clearance for excretion in the kidneys, called the renal clearance, is defined as

$$CL_R = \text{(rate of elimination by excretion in the kidneys)} \ / \ C$$

while the clearance for elimination by metabolism in the liver, called the hepatic clearance, is defined as

$$CL_H = \text{(rate of elimination by hepatic metabolism)}/C$$

Since the total rate of elimination is the sum of the rates for the various routes, and the arterial plasma concentration in the definitions is the same, the partial clearances add to give a total, whole-body or systemic clearance,

$$CL = CL_R + CL_H + ...$$

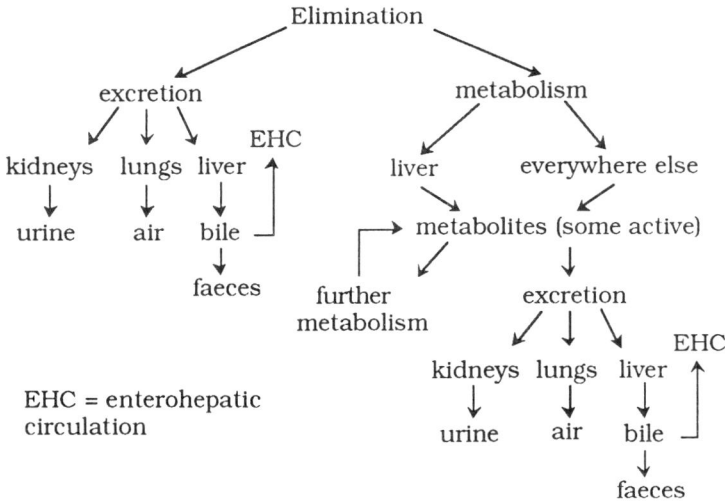

Figure 2.4 Routes of elimination. A drug has been eliminated from the body when it has been excreted or metabolized to some other form. Excretion of unchanged drugs occurs primarily in the kidneys; metabolism primarily in the liver. The metabolites are often but not always inactive. Substances secreted into the bile by the liver can be reabsorbed from the intestines leading to enterohepatic circulation (EHC) (see Section 5.1).

3   RENAL EXCRETION

The kidneys eliminate substances from the body by excreting them in the urine. The mechanisms which determine the rate of this excretion are described as filtration, secretion, and reabsorption (see Fig. 3.1).

3.1   FILTRATION

In the glomeruli about one-fifth of the volume of plasma arriving from the arteries is filtered into the tubules while the rest leaves via the efferent arterioles. **Any dissolved solute smaller than about the size of haemoglobin, and thus any drug in a free form, is**

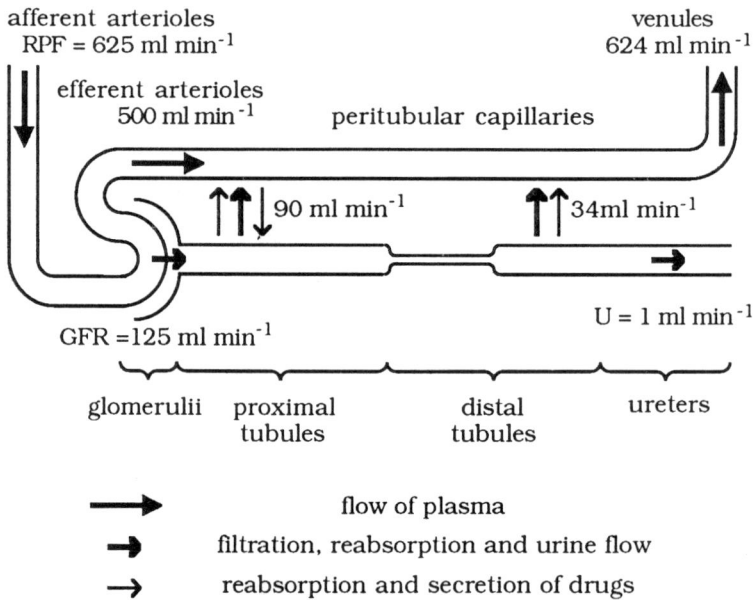

Figure 3.1 A schematic renal tubule with its associated blood vessels. The total values for both kidneys are indicated for renal plasma flow, RPF; glomerular filtration rate, GFR; urine flow rate, U; and the rates of fluid reabsorption. Most of the filtered water, sodium chloride and sodium bicarbonate is reabsorbed. Drugs can be secreted or reabsorbed by specific mechanisms in the proximal tubules. Passive reabsorption of lipid soluble drugs occurs along the entire tubule.

filtered in the same proportion as the water. The free concentrations of filtered drugs are the same in the filtrate, the remaining plasma, and the plasma that arrived at the glomerulus. By contrast almost all the plasma proteins, blood cells, and bound drug both enter and leave in the blood flow. The concentrations in the efferent arterioles of both the binding sites for drugs and the bound drugs are about 20% higher than in the afferent arterioles. These changes together with the lack of change in the free concentration preserve the equilibrium between bound and free drug with no difference between the amount of bound drug arriving at and leaving the glomerulus in the blood.

For small substances **the properties of glomerular filtration can be summarized as**

$$\text{filtration rate of a substance} = \text{GFR} \cdot C^{\text{free}}$$

where C^{free} is the free concentration of the substance in arterial plasma and GFR is the glomerular filtration rate, conventionally taken to be $125\,\text{ml}\,\text{min}^{-1}$ or $1.8\,\text{ml}\,\text{min}^{-1}\text{kg}^{-1}$. If a filtered substance cannot be reabsorbed across the tubule wall, then all that is filtered will be excreted. If there is also no secretion, the renal clearance will be

$$CL_R = \frac{\text{excretion}}{C} = \frac{\text{filtration}}{C} = \frac{\text{GFR} \cdot C^{\text{free}}}{C}$$

Because C^{free}/C can't be greater than 1, the maximum clearance possible by this mechanism equals the GFR. **Substances that are eliminated primarily by glomerular filtration are polar or charged and have little binding to plasma proteins.** Examples of drugs eliminated by this mechanism include the aminoglycosides, atenolol, flucytosine, lithium (partially reabsorbed), and vancomycin.

The clearance of inulin calculated as (rate of elimination)/C_{ss} is used in experimental work for measurement of GFR. Inulin is ideal for this purpose because it is freely filtered, neither secreted nor reabsorbed, non-toxic, easily measured, and eliminated only by renal excretion. However, it is rarely used clinically because it must be injected or infused while another suitable substance, creatinine, is present naturally. The use of creatinine clearance is discussed in Section 3.5.

3.2   SECRETION

Substances can be extracted from plasma and secreted into the proximal tubules by the cells which make up the tubular wall. Many weak acids and organic anions can compete with each other for secretion by one system, while weak bases and organic cations compete for another. Substrates for the first include many foreign molecules that have been conjugated in the liver (see Section 4.2 and Chapter 5), *p*-aminohippuric acid, salicylate, uric acid, methotrexate, diuretics like frusemide and the thiazides, and many penicillins. Basic or cationic substrates include cimetidine, creatinine, histamine, choline and hexamethonium.

Secretion of a substance into the tubule lowers the free concentration of the substance in the plasma which reduces the rate at which free molecules bind to the plasma proteins. The rate of dissociation then exceeds the rate of binding which reduces the amount of the substance bound and partially replaces the free molecules that were secreted. **If the secretion is fast enough and the free fraction large enough,** the newly released drug is also secreted and **the process continues until virtually all of the drug arriving in the blood plasma, both free and bound, has been extracted.** Substances that are eliminated by secretion are usually too polar to cross cell membranes rapidly except by a specific mechanism, and thus any of the drug that enters the kidneys within blood cells cannot escape quickly enough to be secreted. **The maximum renal clearance for a drug that is rapidly secreted and not reabsorbed approaches**

$$CL_R = \frac{\text{rate of secretion + filtration}}{C}$$

$$= \frac{\text{rate at which it arrives in the plasma}}{C}$$

$$= \frac{RPF \cdot C}{C} = RPF$$

Renal plasma flow (RPF) is usually taken as 625 ml min^{-1} or 8.9 ml min^{-1} kg^{-1}. The clearance of the marker substance *p*-aminohippuric acid is used to measure renal plasma flow. For substances eliminated primarily by secretion, changes in the percentage bound in plasma have little effect on the total clearance.

3.3   REABSORPTION AND FACTORS THAT LIMIT RENAL EXCRETION

Many substances cannot be excreted efficiently by the kidneys. Some never enter the tubules in sufficient quantities. Their free fraction in plasma is too small for significant filtration and they are not secreted. Others that are sufficiently lipid-soluble enter the tubules but are extensively reabsorbed.

As fluid passes along the tubules, sodium, chloride, bicarbonate, many other substances, and water are reabsorbed, leaving behind less than 1% of the fluid to be excreted as the urine. **Solutes whose reabsorption lags behind that of water** are therefore carried in a smaller and smaller volume of fluid, i.e. they **become more concentrated in the tubular fluid.** Because the rate of excretion is equal to both $CL_R C$ and $C_{ur} U$, where C_{ur} is the concentration in urineand U is the urine flow rate,

$$CL_R = \frac{C_{ur}}{C} U$$

A large renal clearance is possible only if the total concentration in urine is much larger than the total concentration in plasma. For example the clearance of penicillin G is about $550\,ml\,min^{-1}$. With a plasma concentration of $10\,\mu g\,ml^{-1}$ and a urine flow rate of $1\,ml\,min^{-1}$, the concentration in urine will be $10\cdot550/1 = 5.5\,mg\,ml^{-1}$.

Reabsorption of drugs in the distal tubules occurs down the concentration gradient between tubular fluid and plasma. For any substance that is sufficiently lipid-soluble to diffuse rapidly across the membranes of the tubular wall, reabsorption is extensive and the concentration in the tubule barely rises above the free concentration in the plasma. The renal clearance is then typically less than the urine flow rate, $1\,ml\,min^{-1}$ $(0.015\,ml\,min^{-1}\,kg^{-1})$. The kidneys are rarely the main route for elimination when the renal clearance is this small.

Many drugs that can be absorbed from the intestines are sufficiently lipid-soluble to cross cell membranes rapidly. With the exception of a few weak bases (see below) **these are easily reabsorbed and are poorly eliminated by the kidneys. Even freely filtered drugs like paracetamol and ethanol are excreted very slowly. By contrast conjugated drug metabolites** (see Section 4.2) **are excreted because most are filtered, many are avidly secreted and few are reabsorbed.**

3.4 EXCRETION OF WEAK ACIDS AND BASES

Many drugs are weak acids or bases that can exist in both neutral and charged forms (for extensive lists see Bowman & Rand, pp. 40.4 and 40.5). The charged forms usually cannot cross the walls of the distal tubule. However, association and dissociation reactions for weak acids and bases are very rapid, and the concentrations of the charged and neutral forms will remain at equilibrium with each other. If the neutral form can cross the wall, as the tubular fluid is reabsorbed and tubular concentrations increase, some of the neutral form will escape. Therefore, its concentration in the tubule will increase less than the concentration of the charged form, some of the charged form will be converted to the neutral form to preserve the equilibrium between forms, and indirectly the charged form will also escape.

For some weak acids and bases including frusemide, the thiazides, many penicillins, and methotrexate, **reabsorption is slow either because there is too little of the neutral form to allow appreciable absorption or because both the charged and neutral forms can't cross the tubule wall. For these drugs the rate of renal excretion is determined primarily by the rates of filtration and secretion** and urine flow rate has virtually no effect on elimination.

For many other weak acids and bases, the neutral form crosses the tubule wall sufficiently rapidly for the concentrations of the neutral form in urine and plasma to approach equilibrium with each other. As long as this equilibrium is maintained, the renal clearance is usually small and it is proportional to the urine flow rate,

$$CL_R = \frac{C_{ur}}{C} U = \frac{(\text{charged + neutral})_{urine}}{(\text{charged + neutral + bound})_{plasma}} U$$

Because the free concentrations of the neutral form in plasma and urine are almost the same, for a large clearance the concentration of the charged form in urine must be much larger than both the free concentration of the neutral form and the free concentration of the charged form in the plasma. (In addition the concentration of the charged form must be much larger than the concentration of any bound form in plasma).

The equilibrium between the charged and neutral forms of a weak base in urine (see Fig. 3.2) can be described by its dissociation constant,

urine | plasma

$$B_{ur} \rightleftharpoons B_p$$

$$+ \qquad +$$

$$H^+_{ur} \qquad H^+_p$$

$$\Updownarrow \qquad \Updownarrow$$

$$BH^+_{ur} \qquad BH^+_p$$

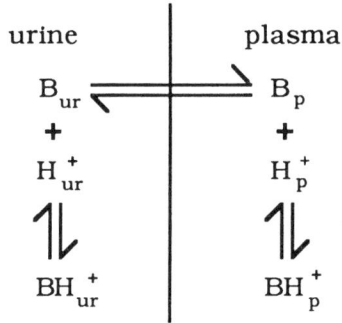

Figure 3.2 The equilibria between the charged and neutral forms of a weak base whose neutral form is easily reabsorbed. The concentration of the cationic form can be much higher in the urine than in plasma if the hydrogen ion concentration is also much greater (see text). In effect the weak base is "trapped" in the low pH medium by conversion to a charged form.

$$K = \frac{H^+_{ur} B_{ur}}{BH^+_{ur}}$$

where BH^+_{ur} and B_{ur} are the concentrations of the charged and neutral forms in urine. This equation can be converted to the Henderson-Hasselbalch equation by taking logs and using the normal definitions for pH and pK,

$$pH = -\log[H^+]$$

and

$$pK = -\log[K]$$

with the result

$$pH_{ur} = pK + \log \left[\frac{B_{ur}}{BH^+_{ur}} \right]$$

Similarly for a weak acid,

$$pH_{ur} = pK + \log \left[\frac{A^-_{ur}}{AH_{ur}} \right]$$

Thus the condition that most of the drug in urine must be in the charged form requires $pH_{ur} < pK$ for a weak base and $pH_{ur} > pK$ for a weak acid.

Equilibrium with the same dissociation constant exists in both plasma and urine, i.e. for a weak base

$$K = \frac{H^+_{ur} B_{ur}}{BH^+_{ur}} = \frac{H^+_p B_p}{BH^+_p}$$

Thus the condition that the concentration of the charged form must be greater in the urine than in plasma requires $H_{ur}^+ > H_p^+$, i.e. $pH_{ur} < pH_p$ for a weak base and $H_{ur}^+ < H_p^+$, i.e. $pH_{ur} > pH_p$ for a weak acid.

When urine pH is more than 2 units below plasma pH a large renal clearance is possible for a weak base with pK > 7 even if the neutral form is permeant. Weak bases whose total clearance is affected by urine pH and flow rate include amphetamine and ephedrine. Recovery from overdoses of amphetamine can be hastened by forcing a diuresis and administering NH_4Cl to make the urine acid.

Urine pH is usually less than plasma pH, 7.4, and never rises much above 8.4. Thus **for a weak acid whose neutral form is highly permeant, the renal clearance is small**. Even so, in the treatment of salicylate or barbiturate poisoning the renal clearance can be made significant by administering sodium bicarbonate and a diuretic to increase urinary pH and force a diuresis.

An example of the effect of pH when the neutral form has intermediate permeability across the tubule wall is provided by the oral hypoglycaemic drug, chlorpropamide. The neutral form of this weak acid is permeant but not highly so. For urine pH below 5, most of the drug in the distal tubules is neutral, it is reabsorbed and less than 10% of a dose is excreted by the kidneys. The clearance is small, $0.02\,ml\,min^{-1}kg^{-1}$, and occurs via metabolism in the liver. For urine pH above 7, too little of the drug is neutral to allow sufficiently rapid reabsorption, the clearance is about four times larger, and more than 80% of a dose is excreted by the kidneys.

3.5   THE USE OF CREATININE CLEARANCE TO ADJUST DOSE RATES

If the clearance of a drug changes, either the dose rate must be altered or the average concentration will change. Two fold reductions in renal clearances are commonly seen even in healthy persons over 65, and much larger changes occur in renal failure. Normally the clearance is reduced in the same proportion for a variety of drugs and for substances used as markers. Similarly renal clearances of many substances are increased in the obese.

Because renal clearances for many drugs and markers change in parallel, the change in renal function measured using a marker can be used to adjust the dose rates for drugs. The measure of renal function used most often for this purpose is the clearance of creatinine. Creatinine is a waste product of normal muscle metabolism. The muscles effectively infuse it into the circulation at a nearly constant rate and the kidneys excrete it primarily by filtration. Both its plasma concentration and the amount in the urine can be measured relatively easily, and its renal clearance can be calculated using the normal relation

$$CL_{Cr} = \frac{\text{rate of creatinine excretion}}{C_{Cr}}$$

There is some secretion of creatinine and some error in the determination of the plasma concentration. Nevertheless the values of CL_{Cr} closely parallel the values of GFR.

The use of creatinine in the adjustment of the dose rate of a drug is based on the experimentally determined relation between the clearance of the drug and CL_{Cr}. For instance for the aminoglycoside antibiotic, gentamicin, the relation is given as, (Goodman & Gilman, p. 1688)

$$CL = 0.73 \cdot CL_{Cr} + 0.06 \, \text{ml min}^{-1} \, \text{kg}^{-1}$$

with CL and CL_{Cr} both expressed in the units $\text{ml min}^{-1} \text{kg}^{-1}$. For a 70 kg man this equation can be rewritten as

$$CL = 0.73 \cdot CL_{Cr} + 4.2 \, \text{ml min}^{-1}$$

with both clearances in ml min^{-1}. The second numerical constant in these relations presumably represents non-renal elimination.

To avoid toxic effects in the kidneys, the inner ears, and the vestibular apparatus, the average concentration of gentamicin must not be allowed to exceed about $4 \, \mu\text{g ml}^{-1}$. Using the tabulated relation between the gentamicin and creatinine clearances, an average plasma concentration of $4 \, \mu\text{g ml}^{-1}$ and a normal creatinine clearance of $120 \, \text{ml min}^{-1}$, corresponds to a dose rate $DR = CL \cdot C_{av} = 4 \cdot (120 \cdot 0.73 + 4.2) = 370 \, \mu\text{g min}^{-1}$. With moderate renal failure and a creatinine clearance of $40 \, \text{ml min}^{-1}$, the dose rate for $4 \, \mu\text{g ml}^{-1}$ would be $4 \cdot (40 \cdot 0.73 + 4.2) = 135 \, \mu\text{g min}^{-1}$. If the higher dose rate were used, the average concentration would be $4 \cdot (370/135) = 11 \, \mu\text{g ml}^{-1}$ which would lead to severe toxicity possibly including permanent deafness.

4 DRUG METABOLISM

Most drugs are not excreted directly; they are eliminated by metabolism. Often there is more than one metabolic pathway leading to a variety of products each of which can be therapeutic, toxic or inactive. Thus when a drug is administered metabolism not only affects the time course of the effects produced it can even determine their nature. The study of the mechanisms of drug metabolism is a major field in experimental pharmacology. Its relative importance is far greater than the space allowed here might suggest. More complete accounts and details for specific drugs can be found in the general references.

Drug metabolism is usually thought of as being divided into two phases. Phase one reactions degrade or modify substrates often converting them into substances that are substrates for phase two. Phase two reactions, called conjugations, attach endogenous groups to suitable sites.

4.1 PHASE ONE METABOLISM

Phase one reactions fall into three general categories, oxidations, reductions, and hydrolyses. Hydrolysis breaks ester and amide bonds: examples include the rapid metabolism of procaine by cholinesterase in plasma and of aspirin to salicylate by esterases mainly in the gut and liver. **Reductions convert the azo linkage, -N=N-, and nitro groups, $-NO_2$, to amines, $-NH_2$.** In addition the quinine group in cytotoxic drugs like doxorubicin and mitomycin C is reduced to the active semi-quinone free radical.

Most phase one reactions are oxidations, many performed by the mixed function oxygenases located in the smooth endoplasmic reticulum of the hepatocytes. When liver cells are homogenized to allow biochemical studies the smooth endoplasmic reticulum is broken up into vesicles called microsomes. The mixed function oxygenases are therefore sometimes called microsomal enzymes. Examples of the reactions they mediate are given in Table 4.1.

The liver receives most of its blood flow from the intestines via the hepatic portal vein. The fact that the drug metabolizing microsomal enzymes are primarily located here suggests that they may have evolved as a means of protecting the body from toxic foreign substances absorbed from the diet. Different but related mixed function oxygenases in the adrenal glands hydroxylate cholesterol in the synthesis of steroid hormones.

As befits a system that metabolizes foreign substances, **the hepatic mixed function oxygenases are remarkably non-selective. The main requirement is that a substrate must be sufficiently non-polar, presumably because it must diffuse into or across membranes to reach the active sites. Substrates that reach the active sites bind to one of a family of cytochromes P_{450},** so called because their complexes with carbon monoxide absorb light near 450nm. Many substrates can be oxidized at more than one position. Normally each oxidation produces a product more polar than the substrate which tends to limit the number of oxidations that occur on any one molecule.

The defining feature of a mixed function oxygenase is the introduction of a single oxygen atom into the substrate by reactions requiring both molecular oxygen and the reducing agent, NADPH. A single pass through this system leads to only one of two ends. Either a single oxygen atom is introduced into the structure,

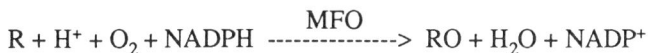

$$R + H^+ + O_2 + NADPH \xrightarrow{\text{MFO}} RO + H_2O + NADP^+$$

or an alkyl side chain is replaced by a hydrogen atom, for example

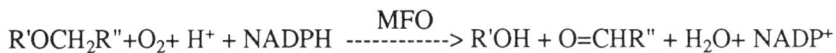

$$R'OCH_2R'' + O_2 + H^+ + NADPH \xrightarrow{\text{MFO}} R'OH + O=CHR'' + H_2O + NADP^+$$

Note that even in dealkylation a single oxygen atom has been introduced into the original structure, it's just that the oxygen is now part of the side chain that has been removed.

As indicated in Fig. 4.1, the relatively simple stoichiometry given above hides considerable ignorance about the actual mechanisms and even about the identity of some of the participants. While there appears to be only one type of cytochrome P_{450} reductase, there are a number of related cytochromes P_{450} with different but overlapping substrate specificities.

Table 4.1 Examples of microsomal oxidations
(An arrow indicates the oxygen introduced by the mixed
function oxygenases)

(a) Aliphatic hydroxylation

Example: pentobarbitone

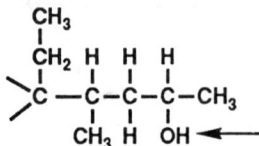

(b) Aromatic hydroxylation

Example: phenytoin

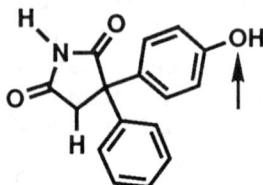

(c) Formation of epoxides

Example: benzanthracene

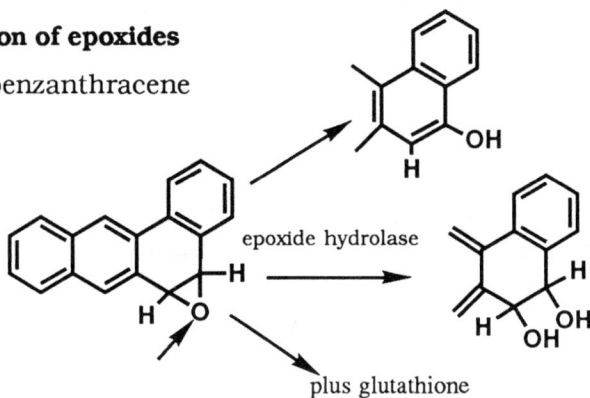

epoxide hydrolase

plus glutathione

Most epoxides are rapidly converted to alcohols and diols. Two
oxidations can form diol-epoxides (see Fig.4.4).

(d) Dealkylation

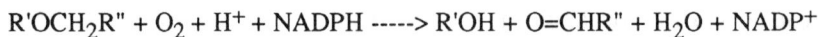

R'OCH$_2$R" + O$_2$ + H$^+$ + NADPH -----> R'OH + O=CHR" + H$_2$O + NADP$^+$

Example:

phenacetin   to   paracetamol

R,R'NCH$_2$R" + O$_2$ + H$^+$+ NADPH ---> R,R'NH + O=CHR" + H$_2$O + NADP$^+$

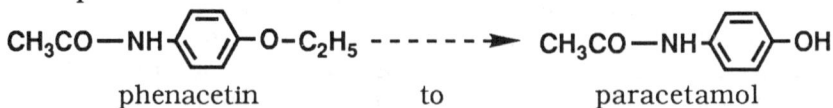

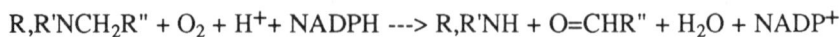

Example: diazepam to desmethyldiazepam

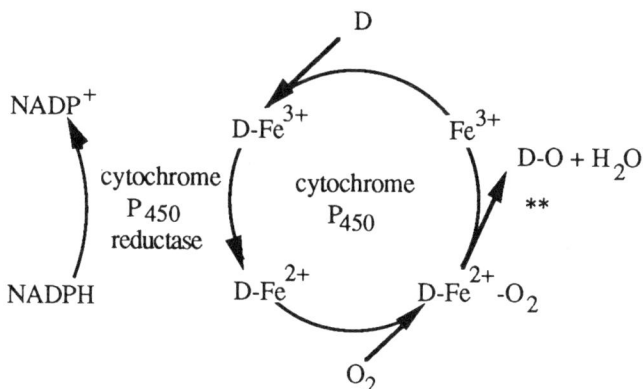

Figure 4.1 A schematic indication of the the oxidation of a drug, D, by a mixed function oxygenase. The drug and molecular oxygen both bind to the iron atom within the haem of a cytochrome P_{450}. The substrate binds to the oxidized form. The iron in the complex is then reduced from Fe^{3+} to Fe^{2+} by cytochrome P_{450} reductase. The reduced complex then takes up oxygen which oxidizes both the iron and the substrate. Somehow at the stage marked ** a second electron is donated, one oxygen is inserted into the substrate and the other oxygen is transferred to two H^{+} atoms.

Some foreign molecule oxidations are not the work of the cytochrome P_{450} system. Examples include reactions catalysed by the cytoplasmic enzymes alcohol dehydrogenase and aldehyde dehydrogenase, and the mitochondrial family of monoamine oxidases that oxidize amines to aldehydes.

4.2 PHASE TWO METABOLISM

Examples of phase two reactions are given in Table 4.2. **Suitable sites for conjugation or attachment of endogenous groups include**

Table 4.1 continued

The products of phase one oxidations are often substrates for conjugations. Other reactions that can be mediated by mixed function oxygenases include: sulphoxidation, S ---> S=O, as for chlorpromazine; desulphuration, =S ---> =O, as for parathion to paraoxon and thiopentone to pentobarbitone; oxidative deamination, $R-CH(CH_3)-NH_2$ ---> $R-C(CH_3)=O + NH_3$, as for amphetamine to phenylacetone; and N-hydroxylation leading to hydroxylamines (see Fig. 4.3).

Table 4.2 Phase two reactions: conjugations

(a) Glucuronidation: Glucuronic acid can be transferred from uridine diphosphate (UDP) to hydroxyls, carboxyls, aromatic amines, etc. to form the glucuronide, e.g.

ROH + UDPglucuronide ---> UDP$^-$ + H$^+$ +

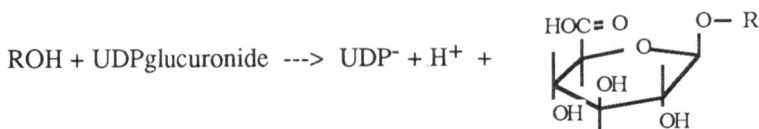

Natural substrates include bilirubin and steroid hormones hydroxylated by phase one metabolism. This conjugation is microsomal. It is inducible by phenobarbitone. The others are non-microsomal.

(b) Sulphation: Sulphate can be transferred by sulphotransferases from adenosine 5'-phosphosulphate to hydroxyl groups and amines.

(c) Acylation (usually acetylation): The acyl group is transferred from Acyl-CoA to acceptors, e.g. aromatic amines;.
Examples: procainamide, isoniazid.

(d) Conjugation with glycine: Substances with a free carboxyl that can be linked to Co-A can then be transferred to the amine of various amino acids--most often glycine.

benzoic acid   hippuric acid

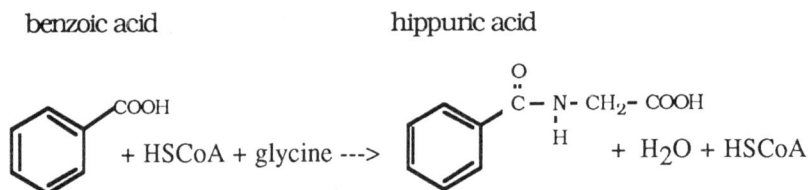

(e) Methylation: A methyl group can be transferred from S-adenosyl methionine. N-, O-, and S- methylations occur but primarily of endogenous substrates, e.g. noradrenaline to normetanephrine.

(f) Conjugation with glutathione: Glutathione complexes with epoxides, thus preventing the formation of diol-epoxides. Exhaustion of the supply of glutathione is a mechanism which might produce a threshold level for the carcinogenic action of aromatic ring compounds.

hydroxyls, carboxyls, amines, and sulphonamides. Groups which can be attached include glucuronide, sulphate, acetate, glycine and others. Most conjugates are pharmacologically inactive. (Notable exceptions are N-acetylprocainamide and morphine-6-gluconate.) Usually conjugates are sufficiently polar that they cannot undergo phase one reactions but can be excreted by filtration and concentration in the urine. Many are avidly secreted into urine or bile (see Section 3.2 and Chapter 5).

4.3 GENETIC VARIATION IN DRUG METABOLISM

Most drugs are eliminated by more than one route and thus their metabolism may be controlled by several enzymes under the control of different genes (polygenic inheritance). Even the complete absence of one of these enzymes may go undetected as the elimination of the drug can still proceed by other routes. In a large population whose members have different combinations of variant genes, the observed clearances will be spread over a single continuous range (see Fig. 4.2). By contrast for a few drugs, change at a single gene locus can dramatically alter elimination (monogenic inheritance). There are then distinct groups in the population with higher or lower clearances (see Fig. 4.2). Several examples are listed in Table 4.3. If the alternative gene produces an inactive enzyme, there will usually be two groups, those who do and those who do not have a copy of the normal gene.

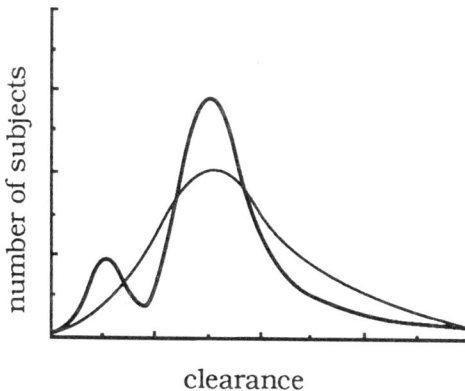

Figure 4.2 The number of members of a population observed to clear a drug at various rates. The heavier curve represents a bimodal distribution like that observed for acetylation of isoniazid; the lighter curve a unimodal distribution as observed for many drugs.

Table 4.3 Examples of genetic variability in drug metabolism

Enzyme affected	Characteristic drugs	Effect
Plasma cholinesterase	Suxamethonium	Decreased rate of hydrolysis leading to increased duration of neuromuscular junction blockade
N-acetyltransferase	Isoniazid Procainamide Sulphonamides	Decreased rate of acetylation leading to high concentrations and toxicity (isoniazid) or prolonged effects (procainamide)
A mixed function oxygenase mediating aromatic hydroxylation	Debrisoquine	40-fold difference in dose requirements for antihypertensive effect
(This defect is closely related to impaired metabolism of phenytoin, phenacetin, propranolol, and nortriptyline.)		
Alcohol dehydrogenase	Ethanol	Prolonged period of intoxication
Glucose-6-phosphate dehydrogenase deficiency	Many including antimalarials aspirin sulphonamides	Drug induced depletion of NADPH which produces haemolysis and porphyria

4.4 CHANGES IN DRUG METABOLISM WITH DISEASE AND AGE

Liver function and the ability of the liver to metabolize drugs are impaired in the neonate and the aged and also by cirrhosis or acute hepatitis. These changes can alter the clearance of a drug if its rate of elimination is limited by the rate of metabolism (see

Section 5.3). However, it is difficult to give general rules because there is no simple pattern of impairment. For instance the metabolism of phenytoin, chlordiazepoxide, phenylbutazone, and propranolol is reduced in the aged, that of diazepam and nitrazepam is not, while the metabolism of both diazepam and chlordiazepoxide is reduced in cirrhosis. At present the only satisfactory approach is to record the significant changes that occur for each drug. Drugs that are metabolized so rapidly that the liver can process all of the drug that arrives in the hepatic blood flow are discussed in Section 5.4.

4.5 INHIBITION AND INDUCTION OF DRUG METABOLISM

The rate of metabolism of a drug can be increased or decreased by drugs and foreign substances. There are a number of possible mechanisms for inhibition including competition between substrates for the active site, product inhibition, and less specific effects. SKF 525A has as its major action a long-lasting inhibition of the microsomal oxidation of many substrates. Non-microsomal systems can also be inhibited. Examples include the inhibition of monoamine oxidase by antidepressants like tranylcypromine, of xanthine oxidase by allopurinol in the treatment of gout, and of aldehyde dehydrogenase by disulfiram.

Many substances can increase the rate of microsomal drug metabolism by increasing the amount of the metabolic enzymes present. Inducers include barbiturates phenytoin, phenyl-butazone, rifampicin, ethanol (chronic), chlorinated insecticides, cigarette smoke, polycyclic aromatic hydrocarbons, and many others. In simplified terms they fall into two broad groups, the polycyclic aromatic hydrocarbons, which are typified by 3-methylcholanthrene, and the rest, the most studied of which is phenobarbitone. The polycyclic aromatic hydrocarbons induce an increased amount of the particular enzymes responsible for their own metabolism (a type of cytochrome P_{450}). By contrast phenobarbitone induces an increase in the amount of all microsomal systems accompanied by substantial increases in both liver weight and liver blood flow.

Some drugs, including phenobarbitone, can induce their own metabolism leading to an increase in the clearance for subsequent doses. To achieve the same concentrations after induction as before, larger doses must be given.

Although the effects of enzyme inductionand inhibition on rates of metabolism can be dramatic, the consequences are clinically important for only a few drugs. **For inhibition or induction to have significant clinical consequences the affected drug must satisfy three conditions:**

(1) **It must be in clinical use.**

(2) **Its plasma concentration must be critical, i.e. there must be only a narrow range of concentrations in which the drug is both effective and safe,.**

(3) **Its clearance and plasma concentration must be altered sufficiently by induction or inhibition to produce either a reduction in therapeutic effect or the onset of toxicity.**

The drugs which have been implicated as satisfying these conditions are **anticoagulants, like dicoumarol and warfarin, anticonvulsants, like phenytoin and phenobarbitone, and oral hypoglycaemic agents like tolbutamide. In addition contraceptive failure has followed increased steroid metabolism induced by rifampicin.**

A notorious example of enzyme induction was the increased metabolism of anticoagulants that occurred when anticoagulant when administered concurrently with barbiturates. The barbiturate substantially increased the clearance of the anticoagulant and hence the dose rate required to prevent clotting. When subsequently the patients stopped taking the barbiturates, the anticoagulant clearance fell, the plasma concentration increased and the patients were at risk of bleeding to death.

Clinically notable examples of inhibition include the effect of sulphonamide antibiotics on the metabolism of the oral hypoglycaemic agent tolbutamide and the inhibition of phenytoin and warfarin metabolism by the histamine H2 blocker cimetidine used in the treatment and prophylaxis of peptic ulcers.

4.6 METABOLITES AND PRODRUGS

A prodrug is an inactive substance that is metabolized to an active drug. For instance indanyl carbenicillin and carfecillin which are well absorbed after oral doses but inactive are metabolized to carbenicillin, which is an active antibiotic but poorly absorbed. Enalapril is a prodrug for enalaprilate. **Much more commonly it is found that both the drug administered and its metabolites have important effects. A complete pharmacokinetic description of a drug includes description of the activity and fate of all its metabolites.** The importance of metabolites is clearly illustrated by the benzodiazepines. For instance half a dose of flurazepam is metabolized within 2-3 hr to desalkyl flurazepam which is active. Because the time taken for half the desalkyl flurazepam to be eliminated is c. 50 hr, its effects far outlast the presence of flurazepam in the body. The benzodiazepines also illustrate that a substance can undergo a chain of conversions, e.g. diazepam (active) can be N-demethylated to desmethyldiazepam (active) which can be converted by aliphatic hydroxylation to oxazepam (active). Finally this compound is inactivated by glucuronide formation. All elements of this chain circulate in plasma, i.e. they can all get in and out of the hepatocytes. A small selection of examples of active metabolites are listed in Table 4.4.

Activation by metabolism is also very important in toxicology. For instance the hepatic damage caused by overdose

Table 4.4 Examples of active metabolites

Drug	Metabolite
Amitriptyline	Nortriptyline
Aspirin	Salicylate
Chlordiazepoxide	Desmethylchlordiazepoxide Demoxepam Desmethyldiazepam
Cortisone	Cortisol
Haloperidol	Dihydrohaloperidol
Imipramine	Desmethylimipramine
Lignocaine	Monoethylglycinexylidide Glycinexylidide
Morphine	Morphine-6-gluconate
Phenacetin	Paracetamol
Procainamide	N-acetylprocainamide
Trimethadione	Dimethadione

of paracetamol (acetaminophen is a consequence of the small portion of the dose that is *N*-hydroxylated with conversion to *N*-acetylbenzoquinoneimine (see Fig. 4.3). This reactive substance can combine with glutathione or with macromolecules. Hepatic necrosis occurs in paracetamol overdose when *N*-hydroxylation proceeds so rapidly that the supply of glutathione is depleted. Another example of immense practical importance is the metabolism of many polycyclic aromatic hydrocarbons, which are themselves not carcinogens, into diol-epoxides which are (see Fig. 4.4). Polycyclic hydrocarbons are found in soot, smoke (including cigarette smoke) and charcoal-grilled meat. Still more examples of the production of toxic products are the formation of formaldehyde from methanol and the release of fluoride ions from the general anaesthetic methoxyflurane.

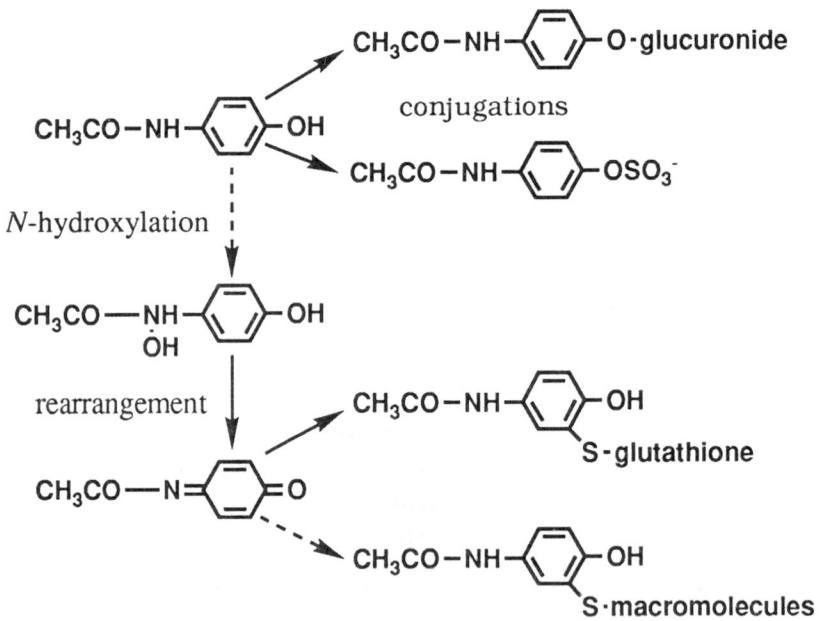

Figure 4.3 Metabolism of paracetamol. Solid arrows indicate the primary routes, the dashed arrows the route which leads to hepatic necrosis. *N*-hydroxylation followed by rearrangement produces *N*-acetylbenzoquinoneimine.

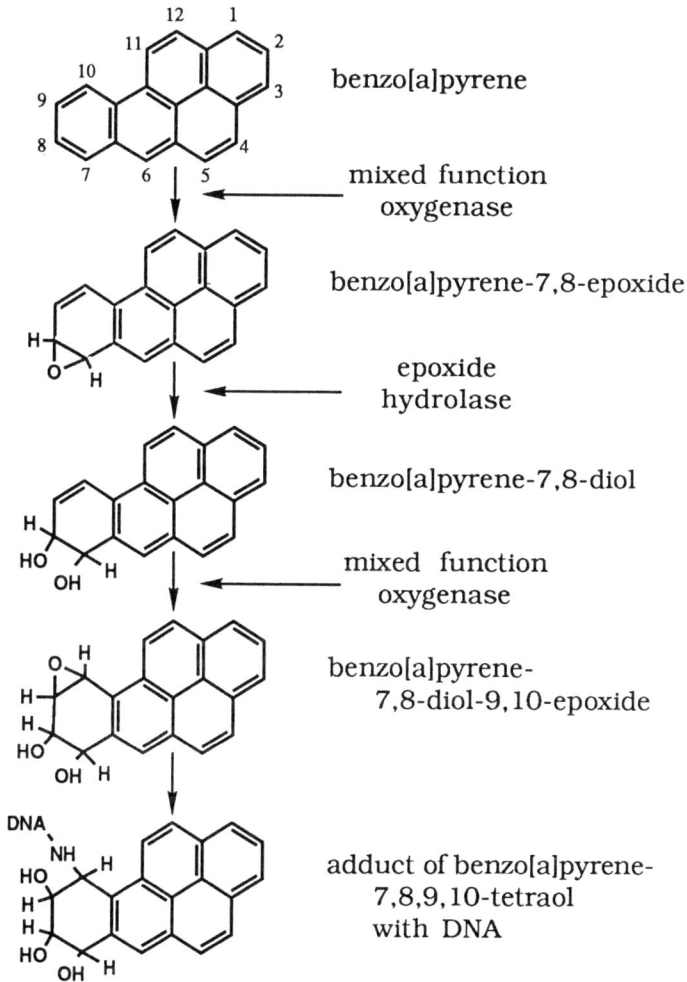

Figure 4.4 The activation of benzo[a]pyrene to a diol-epoxide which is a potent carcinogen as a result of its binding to the adenosine bases of DNA.

5 HEPATIC ELIMINATION

For a drug to be eliminated by the liver it must enter the hepatocytes. From there it can be returned to the blood, secreted into bile, or metabolized (see Figs. 5.1 and 5.2). All lipid-soluble molecules can enter the cells, and there are transporters that facilitate entry of many types of polar molecules.

Secretion of unmodified foreign molecules into the bile is rare, but it is seen with some sulphonamides with large substituents and with indocyanine green (see Section 5.4).

The metabolism of drugs was discussed in the preceding chapter. Products of phase 1 metabolism can be metabolized further, secreted into the bile, or returned to the blood and distributed throughout the body. The fate of conjugates depends on their size. For drugs with molecular weights less than about 300 the conjugates usually re-enter the blood, probably via the same transporters that allow polar molecules to enter the cells. These conjugates are frequently excellent substrates for secretion in the renal tubules. Larger conjugates are primarily secreted into the bile. The mechanism of the secretion is unknown but probably closely related to the mechanism for the secretion of

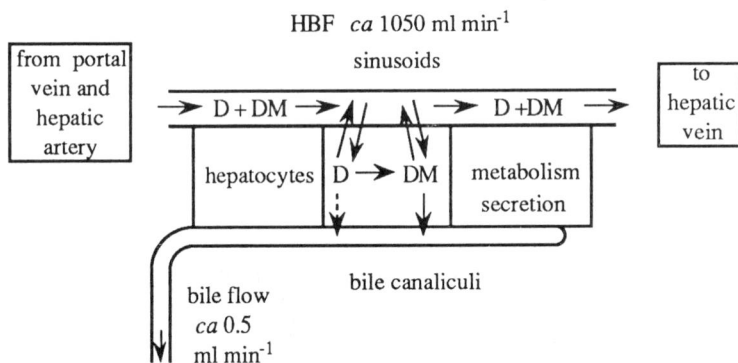

Figure 5.1 Schematic diagram of the relation between the hepatic blood vessels, the hepatocytes, and the bile canaliculi. Drugs, D, as well as metabolites, DM, that have previously entered the blood are brought to the liver by the hepatic blood flow, HBF. There they diffuse or are transported in both directions across the hepatocyte membranes facing the sinusoids. Secretion into the bile canaliculi is irreversible. Within the hepatocytes metabolism reduces the concentration of drug and increases the concentration of metabolites. The metabolites may be more or less active pharmacologically then the original drug.

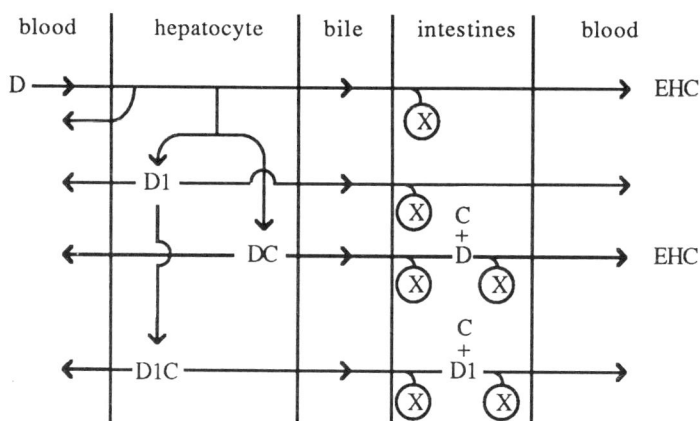

Figure 5.2 Possible fates for a drug which enters a liver hepatocyte. Here D indicates the drug, D1 a product of phase one metabolism, DC and D1C represent conjugates of the drug and metabolite, X indicates excretion, and EHC stands for enterohepatic circulation.

bile salts. Substances secreted into bile usually possess highly polar groups and thus once in the bile they can't escape.

Bile is delivered into the small intestines. There drugs and metabolites can have several different fates (see Fig. 5.2). **They can be excreted; unmodified drug can be reabsorbed; and conjugates can be hydrolysed, releasing the substance that was conjugated.** The substances released can be excreted in the faeces or reabsorbed. Glucuronides are particularly susceptible to hydrolysis.

5.1   ENTEROHEPATIC CIRCULATION

If the substance originally extracted from the blood by the liver is reabsorbed from the intestines into the blood, it has not been eliminated from the body. This movement of a substance from the blood into the liver, then the bile, then the gut, and back to the blood is called the enterohepatic circulation. It performs an important physiological function in the recycling of the bile salts.

A number of drugs are known to be secreted into bile in significant quantities. However, interruption of the enterohepatic circulation by collection of the bile has been part of most studies of biliary secretion and thus these do not directly relate to the rate of drug elimination. There is remarkably little information available about the role of biliary secretion in elimination. For several drugs, including digitoxin (at least in dogs) and diethylstilboestrol, secretion into bile is markedly more rapid than elimination from the body, i.e. there is extensive recirculation.

5.2   EXTRACTION VERSUS CLEARANCE

The rate at which the liver eliminates a drug from the body is described by the metabolic clearance

$$CL = \frac{\text{rate of elimination by metabolism}}{C}$$

However, in discussions of hepatic mechanisms it is more convenient to consider the rate at which the liver extracts the drug from the blood. While extraction and clearance tend to increase or decrease together they are not the same. A drug that is extracted but then reabsorbed via the enterohepatic circulation has not been eliminated. In addition while clearances in tables like those in Goodman & Gilman are based on plasma concentrations, **hepatic extractions are based on concentrations in blood rather than plasma because drugs that are associated with the blood cells are often extracted into the liver. To be metabolized the drugs must be able to enter the hepatocytes, and thus most can also cross blood cell membranes.**

The rate of extraction depends on the intrinsic ability of the liver to deal with the drug and on hepatic blood flow. When entry to the hepatocytes and metabolism are both rapid, the liver extracts all of the drug that arrives in the blood

$$\text{Maximum hepatic extraction rate} = C_{b,A} \, HBF$$

where the hepatic blood flow, HBF, is the sum of the blood flows in the hepatic portal vein and the hepatic artery and $C_{b,A}$ is the concentration when these flows are mixed. The actual rate of extraction is the difference between the rates at which the drug arrives and leaves in the blood, $(C_{b,A} - C_{b,V}) \cdot HBF$ where $C_{b,V}$ is the concentration in the hepatic vein. **The ratio of the actual rate of extraction to the maximum is called the extraction ratio,**

$$E = \frac{(C_{b,A} - C_{b,V}) \cdot HBF}{C_{b,A} HBF} = \frac{(C_{b,A} - C_{b,V})}{C_{b,A}}$$

Put the other way round, the rate of extraction is

$$\text{Rate of extraction} = E \cdot HBF \cdot C_{b,A}$$

When the rate of extraction is limited by the rate at which drug is delivered to the liver, it is said to be blood flow limited. Then by definition everything that arrives is extracted and E approaches 1. Alternatively the rate of extraction can be limited by either the rate at which the drug can enter the hepatocytes or the rate at which it can be metabolized. Then much more arrives than is extracted and E ≪ 1.

If all the extracted drug is eliminated, and both the fraction of the blood volume occupied by cells, H, and the ratio of the concentration in the cells to that in the plasma, C_{rbc}/C, are known, then the clearance can be calculated from the extraction ratio as

$$CL = \frac{(\text{rate of elimination})}{C} = \frac{C_{b,A} E \cdot HBF}{C}$$

$$= \frac{\left[(1 - H) \cdot C + H \cdot C_{rbc}\right] E \cdot HBF}{C}$$

$$= \left[1 + H \cdot \left(\frac{C_{rbc}}{C} - 1\right)\right] \cdot E \cdot HBF$$

When the extraction ratio is nearly 1, the clearance can exceed the hepatic plasma flow if the drug is carried by the blood cells, but even the largest known hepatic clearances, e.g. $1050\,\text{ml min}^{-1}$ for imipramine, are less than hepatic blood flow. (Larger clearances are, of course, possible for drugs cleared in the lungs or at more than one site, e.g. prostacyclin and propofol.)

5.3   EXTRACTION LIMITED BY METABOLISM

If the extraction ratio is small, the concentration of the drug is almost the same in the blood that enters the sinusoid and the blood that leaves, and this concentration is not affected by changes in blood flow. Because the concentration is constant, the rate of drug entry into the hepatocytes is also not affected. Thus for small extraction ratios, when HBF increases, the rate of extraction remains constant, and the extraction ratio E goes down. On the other hand if the ability of the hepatocytes to metabolize or secrete the drug is increased or decreased then the rate of extraction will change. Factors that alter the rate of metabolism include cirrhosis of the liver, age, enzyme induction, and drug interactions (see Sections 4.3 and 4.4). Examples of substances eliminated primarily by the liver but with a low extraction ratio include: chloramphenicol, chlorpromazine, diazepam, digitoxin, paracetamol, phenobarbitone, phenylbutazone, phenytoin, salicylic acid, theophylline, tolbutamide, and warfarin.

5.4   BLOOD FLOW LIMITED EXTRACTION

If the extraction ratio is nearly one, almost all of the drug is extracted from the blood into the hepatocytes and the concentration decreases to low levels as the blood traverses the sinusoids. If the hepatic blood flow is increased and more drug arrives, the average free concentration in the sinusoids will be higher and therefore more drug will be extracted. The extraction ratio remains near one. By contrast because entry into the cells and metabolism are fast enough to extract all the drug, increases or small decreases in these "intrinsic" processes will not produce any change in the actual rate of extraction. Drugs with extraction ratios greater than one half include adrenaline, alprenolol, desmethylimipramine, glyceryl trinitrate, hydrocortisone, imipramine, isoniazid, lignocaine, morphine, naloxone, propranolol and verapamil.

Hepatic blood flow is decreased by standing, exercise, cirrhosis, hepatitis, heart failure and age and it is increased during digestion of a meal. Typically these changes can halve or double the blood flow. At least in principle the effect of a change in flow on the hepatic extraction of substances with high extraction ratios can be measured using a marker substance like indocyanine green and this information used to calculate changes in the elimination of drugs. However, in practice this is rarely done.

Substances absorbed from the stomach or intestines are delivered by the blood to the liver. In the liver, if the extraction ratio is near one, most of the drug is extracted and usually eliminated before it ever reaches the general circulation. This effect, called first pass elimination, is discussed further in Section 6.2.10.

6 ROUTES OF ADMINISTRATION, ABSORPTION AND AVAILABILITY

The processes of elimination, described by the clearance, determine the average rate at which a drug must reach the general circulation to maintain a plasma concentration. The routes of administration and the processes of absorption determine the availability of the doses to the body.

6.1 ROUTES OF ADMINISTRATION

The various routes by which drugs are administered systemically are indicated in Fig. 6.1. Some substances of pharmacological interest, e.g. prostaglandins, are efficiently eliminated by the lungs and thus even when injected intravenously little survives to reach arterial plasma. Substances with such short half-lives are

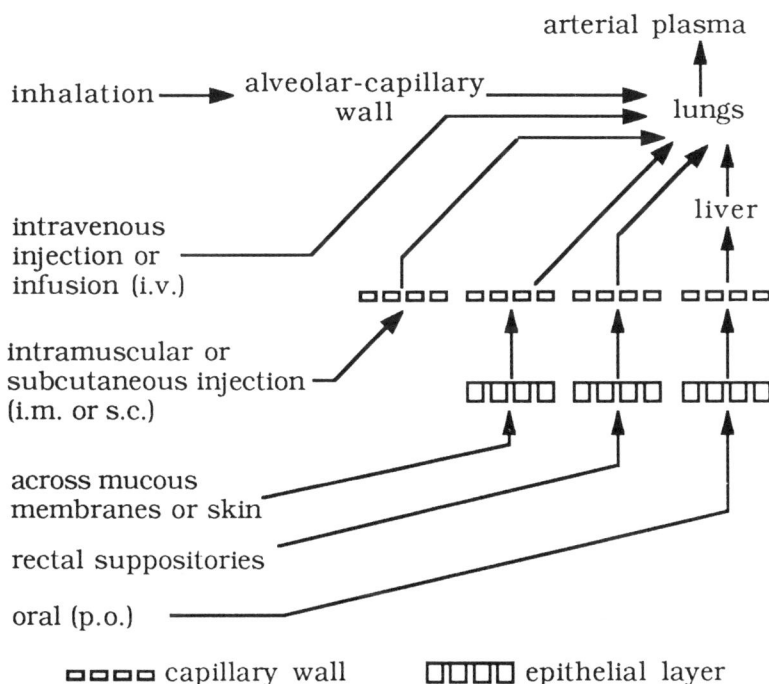

Figure 6.1 Routes of drug administration and the barriers a drug must pass to reach arterial blood plasma.

rarely used as systemically administered drugs. An important exception is the constant infusion of prostacyclin (epoprostenol) to prevent platelet aggregation during renal dialysis.

6.1.1   Intravenous (i.v.) injections and infusions

Intravenous injection has advantages. An accurately known amount of drug reaches the plasma, administration can be very fast and, when the injection or infusion is stopped, no more drug enters the body. The major disadvantages are the skill required of the person administering the dose, the risks involved in producing very high concentrations in the blood at the time of the injection, the high initial rate of elimination which can lead to elimination of a large proportion of the dose in a short time, the risk of infection, and the marked inconvenience to the patient. The high peak concentrations seen with intravenous injection can be avoided by using infusions (see Chapter 9), but this requires cannulation and apparatus to control the rate of infusion.

6.1.2   Intramuscular (i.m.) or subcutaneous (s.c.) injections

Intramuscular or subcutaneous injections deposit the drug in the interstitial fluid of a tissue. This fluid is separated from plasma only by a capillary wall. If it is soluble, the concentration in blood plasma leaving the site will be proportional to the free drug concentration in the local interstitial fluid. Thus drug will be removed from the site and delivered to the body at a rate proportional to the local concentration and the local blood flow. As the local concentration falls so does the rate of delivery. **For drugs that remain in solution following injection, the time for half the drug to be absorbed is variable, but typically 20 to 30 min. Factors affecting the rate include temperature, muscular activity, and gross movement. For many drugs i.m. or s.c. injections provide a reliable means for introducing a known amount of drug into the body without the disadvantages of a large initial peak in concentration (see Fig. 6.3).**

The small volume of fluid in an injection must contain all the drug that is being administered. Thus **typically the drug concentration in the injection medium must be 10,000 to 100,000 times greater than the intended plasma concentration. This high concentration may require that it be dissolved in a special**

solution. If so, it may precipitate when it comes into contact with tissue fluids. For instance weak acids injected as soluble sodium salts in strongly alkaline solution often precipitate when the pH falls to 7.4 in the tissues. Examples of drugs which precipitate after injection include chlordiazepoxide, digoxin, phenytoin, quinidine, and a number of cephalosporins and penicillins.

When precipitation occurs, the free drug concentration at the injection site will depend on the balance between the rate of dissolution and the rate at which the drug diffuses into the blood. **So long as solid remains, the free concentration and the rate at which drug reaches the blood will be roughly constant, i.e. the solid infuses drug into the circulation.** Sustained release or depot preparations deliberately use this effect to produce moderate concentrations for a prolonged period of time. Large crystals of insulin given subcutaneously can produce effects for hours. Similarly penicillin G, procaine and penicillin G benzathine suspensions are used to maintain plasma concentrations over periods ranging from 12 hours to many days.

There are several **disadvantages of intramuscular and subcutaneous injections: high local concentrations of drugs under the skin or in muscles can be damaging; injections can hurt, some quite a lot; there is risk of infection; if precipitation occurs, absorption may be very slow; there is risk that the dose will be administered intravascularly; there can be mechanical damage, e.g. to a nerve; and most injections are given by trained personnel whose time is expensive. Injections are normally used only when oral dosing is not feasible.**

6.1.3   By inhalation

Drug administration by inhalation requires either that the drug be volatile or that it be carried in an extremely fine aerosol or dust. Few drugs are volatile. The obvious exceptions are general anaesthetics (see Chapter 12) and amyl nitrite, which has been used to produce rapid relief of acute angina. Most drugs administered as aerosols or dusts are intended for local application to the airways, e.g. beta-adrenoceptor agonists used for relief of acute asthmatic attacks.

6.1.4   Across the buccal epithelium

Some drugs can be kept in the mouth, usually under the tongue, long enough for a significant amount to be absorbed across the buccal epithelium. One drawback is obvious; many drugs taste horrible. In addition, the need not to swallow until absorption is complete can lead to unpleasant accumulation of saliva. The surface area available for absorption is severely limited and this restricts use of this route to drugs that are sufficiently lipid-soluble to cross the epithelium quickly. Despite these disadvantages a few drugs are given by this route. Sublingual buprenorphine is used to produce postoperative analgesia. Glyceryl trinitrate absorbed from under the tongue is used for rapid relief of acute attacks of angina. If swallowed it is not effective because absorption is too slow and after absorption from the gut it is metabolized in the liver.

6.1.5   Across the skin

Absorption across the skin was until recently regarded as too slow and too unreliable for use. However lipid-soluble drugs and toxic materials can be absorbed if they are kept in contact for a sufficiently long time. This method is now used for several drugs including clonidine and glyceryl trinitrate and is under study for propranolol. It may be appropriate for drugs that must be delivered over a period, are subject to first pass metabolism when given orally, and are sufficiently lipid-soluble.

6.1.6   Rectal

Drugs can be administered rectally in suppositories. The principal advantages of this route are that the venous drainage doesn't go to the liver and absorption can be achieved in patients subject to attacks of vomiting. Promethazine suppositories are used to suppress vomiting. The principal disadvantage of rectal administration is that the rectum is primarily designed for temporary storage, rather than efficient absorption. Absorption rates are often low. For reasons that are obscure, this route of administration is employed more frequently in France than in England.

6.1.7 Oral

Far more drugs are administered orally than by any other route.
Almost anyone can swallow a pill or 5 ml of syrup. Thus oral
medications can be self-administered and a series of doses can be
taken without continuous medical supervision. The savings in
the cost of the time of skilled medical personnel is considerable.
Some oral medications can be added directly to food with obvious
benefits in veterinary practice.

There is another important advantage of oral dosing over
intravenous injection. **Because absorption isn't instantaneous
there is no large initial peak in the plasma concentration (see e.g.
Fig. 6.3).** Thus provided most of the drug is absorbed, at times
sufficiently long after a dose there is actually more of the drug left
in the body from an oral dose than from an intravenous dose.
**Oral dosing can extend the period during which a dose of drug
produces its effects.**

There is a price to be paid for the advantages. Firstly **the other
side of the coin of prolonged action is that the onset of action is
slow. A more important limitation is that the fraction of a dose
that reaches the general circulation is variable and
unpredictable.** The advantages of oral dosing are so substantial
that this route is used even when this fraction is small. The oral
dose is increased above the intravenous dose until the amount
that reaches the general circulation is adequate. Clearly there
must be a limit. In practice, the dose must remain small enough
for the variable amount absorbed never to be too great.

6.2 FACTORS AFFECTING THE ABSORPTION AND AVAILABILITY OF ORALLY ADMINISTERED DRUGS

6.2.1 Disintegration

A drug for oral administration must be presented in a dosage
form that is stable during storage and convenient to swallow. But
the same dosage form must also expose the drug to the fluids in
the gut before it can be absorbed. Some drugs can be administered
as syrups, but many are not sufficiently stable in this form.
Tablets must hold together well while dry, but break apart or
disintegrate rapidly in the gut fluids. **Use of different binders and
fillers to hold the tablets together and give them shape can
produce large variations in the rate and, more importantly, the**

extent of absorption. An infamous example was the increase in the extent of absorption of phenytoin when a manufacturer in Australia changed the binder from calcium sulphate to sodium lactate. Prior to 1969 it was not appreciated that less than half the dose was absorbed from the tablets containing calcium sulphate, and it therefor came as a surprise when patients whose doses had been previously adjusted developed severe toxic symptoms after the change to sodium lactate. The increase in the extent of absorption, as much as two fold, led to phenytoin reaching the body more rapidly than it could be metabolized. Toxicity was then inevitable (see Sections 2.4 and E.2.5).

As an alternative to tablets, capsules can be designed to break down either in the acid conditions of the stomach or the alkaline conditions of the duodenum. Some form of coating is certainly desirable if the drug is really unpleasant to taste. The need to break down the coating or capsule lining can delay absorption, but often to no greater extent than from a tablet (see Section 6.2.6). Sometimes part of a dose is coated so that absorption of the parts occurs at different rates producing a sustained release of the drug (see Chapter 10). Coatings and capsules add to the cost of the drug.

6.2.2   Water solubility, rate of dissolution and particle size

Once the tablet has disintegrated or the capsule coating has dissolved the particles of drug that were formed during manufacture are exposed to the solution. The rate at which the molecules then go into solution increases with the surface area of the particles and with the solubility of the drug. A particle of solid is surrounded by a thin stagnant layer of fluid, sometimes called the unstirred layer or the diffusion layer. The rate-limiting step in dissolving the solid is often diffusion of the molecules across this layer. Right next to the surface of the solid the solution is then saturated. **The higher the saturated concentration of the drug and the larger the surface area of the solid, the faster diffusion and thus dissolution occur.** Large variations in the rate and extent of absorption have been observed for digoxin from tablets with particles milled to different sizes. Large particle sizes can be used deliberately to reduce dissolution and subsequent decomposition of a drug in the acid conditions of the stomach.

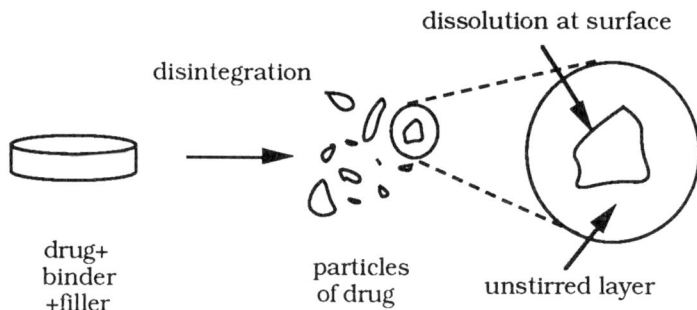

Figure 6.2   The disintegration and dissolution of a tablet. A tablet disintegrates releasing the manufactured particles of the drug. These particles must then dissolve. In many instances the solution immediately adjacent to the surface is nearly saturated and the rate of dissolution is limited by the rate of diffusion across the unstirred layer.

6.2.3   Lipid-solubility

To get from the lumen of the gut to the blood, the drug must cross the epithelium. **Absorption at an appreciable rate usually requires that the substance is sufficiently lipid-soluble to get through cell membranes. Highly polar or charged drugs that are not recognized by one of the specific transport systems, e.g. the aminoglycosides like gentamicin, must be given by injection.**

6.2.4   pH and pK

Many drugs are weak acids or bases possessing both charged and neutral forms. By altering the proportions of these forms, **the pH of the gut fluids can affect both the dissolution of drug particles and the subsequent movement of drug molecules across the gut epithelium.**

The charged forms of most weak acids and bases are more soluble in water than the neutral forms. A pH that favours the charged form at the surface of a drug particle raises the local concentration at this surface which increases the rate of dissolution (see Section 6.2.2). This increase is the theoretical basis for formulating aspirin together with a buffer in order to make the region around the tablet alkaline, though the effect on the overall rate of absorption isn't large.

The tetracyclines provide an important example of the effect of pH on aqueous solubility. At low pH in the stomach these drugs dissolve in a charged form but they precipitate when the intermediate pH in the intestines converts them to a neutral form. Thus any portion that isn't absorbed from the stomach is excreted in the faeces.

The pH at the gut wall can affect the rate and direction of movement across the gut epithelium. Frequently the neutral forms of weak acids or weak bases can cross the epithelium rapidly while the charged forms cannot. However, association and dissociation reactions for weak acids and bases are very rapid, and the concentrations of the charged and neutral forms remain at equilibrium with each other. If the neutral form is absorbed, which lowers its concentration, there will be conversion of the charged to the neutral form maintaining the equilibrium. Even when the concentration of the neutral form is only a small fraction of the total, its continued absorption can lead to virtually total absorption of the drug (compare Section 3.4). Absorption becomes so slow as to be incomplete only when the concentration of the neutral form falls well below 1%. **In the intestines absorption is found to be rapid for either weak acids with pK>3 or weak bases with pK<7.8 provided the neutral forms are readily absorbed. The low pH in the stomach favours absorption of weak acids, though other factors (see Section 6.2.5) determine that absorption still occurs primarily in the intestines. Weak bases are generally not absorbed from the stomach** and for some, e.g. quinine, there is clearly secretion.

Secretion of weak bases into the stomach is predicted by the pH-partition or pH-trapping mechanism discussed in Section 3.4. In plasma perfusing the stomach a fraction of the weak base is in the neutral form. Thus some can cross the stomach wall into the low pH fluid in the lumen. There, unless the pK is very low, virtually all of the weak base will be protonated and trapped. The secreted drug is, of course, delivered to the intestines where it can be reabsorbed.

6.2.5   Surface area of epithelium

Most absorption from the gut occurs in the small intestines because the intestines have much the largest absorptive surface area.

6.2.6   Digestion

For most peptides and proteins digestion prevents the use of the oral route. Insulin is a very important example. Some other drugs are also hydrolysed in acid media. Examples include penicillin G and erythromycin. Erythromycin has been protected from the stomach fluids using tablets with an acid-resisting coating or by enclosing the dose in an acid-resistant capsule. However, until the tablet or capsule leaves the stomach nothing is absorbed. The time for passage to the intestines can vary from 20 min to 8 hr. An alternative strategy is to give the drug as a very coarse powder or as coated granules. There are then many more bits and the arrival in the intestines is more predictable.

6.2.7   Food in the gut

The effect of food can be mechanical or it can involve drug binding. The transit time through the stomach especially for drug particles is both longer and much more variable after a meal than before. This difference can markedly affect the time course of drug absorption and the time required for the onset of effects, e.g. for analgesics. The effects of drug binding to constituents of food are critical for the use of tetracyclines. The tetracylines are soluble and can be absorbed only at low pH and in the absence of high concentrations of calcium and magnesium. After a meal, the pH is normally less acid, and there are a variety of salts present in the stomach. The absorption of tetracyclines can then be substantially depressed, and they can pass on to later portions of the gut with the food and be excreted in the faeces. Other drugs normally taken on an empty stomach because food can reduce their absorption include ampicllin, terbutaline, zidovudine (AZT) and captopril.

Drugs are sometimes given with or after food to minimize gastric irritation or discomfort. Levodopa is thought to produce less central emetic effect when taken after meals.

6.2.8   Vomiting

Vomiting can reduce absorption by expelling part or all of the dose.

6.2.9   Diarrhoea

Absorption can be reduced by diarrhoea if the drug is swept through the intestines before there is sufficient time for it to be absorbed.

6.2.10   First pass effect

Following absorption the drug may be metabolized in the gut wall. The portion that survives is taken by the blood through the hepatic portal vein to the liver where the hepatocytes are the site of metabolism for many drugs (see Section 6.6). The blood then flows via the hepatic vein to the heart. **The portion of the dose that is absorbed from the lumen of the gastro-intestinal tract but eliminated on the way to the heart is said to have undergone first pass elimination.** Drugs for which most of an oral dose is lost in this manner are said to be subject to a **first pass effect** (see Section 5.3). As discussed in the next section, these will have a low availability by the oral route. Drugs and markers which are subject to first pass elimination include adrenaline, alprenolol, bromosulphophthalein, desmethylimipramine, glyceryl trinitrate, hydrocortisone, imipramine, indocyanine green, isoniazid, lignocaine, morphine, naloxone, propranolol, and verapamil. Low but not very low availability may still allow oral administration by using a larger dose provided the availability is not too variable. Millions of patients have taken propranolol orally, even though the fraction that survives the first pass effect can be less than a third.

6.3   AVAILABILITY: THE EXTENT OF DRUG ABSORPTION

The availability of a dosage form, F, is defined as the fraction of a dose that reaches the heart and general circulation. The availability can be substantially less than one for an injection if the drug can be metabolized at the site of injection. It can appear to be very small if a portion of the dose is released so slowly that it produces undetectable concentrations over a prolonged period. Low availability is more common for drugs given orally. It can be a result of poor absorption or of first pass elimination.

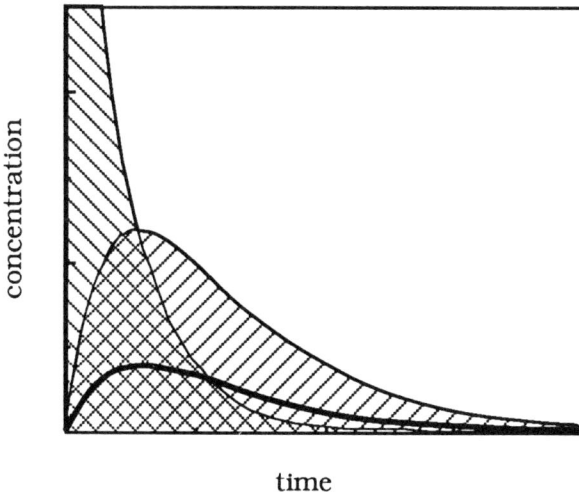

time

Figure 6.3 Comparison of plasma concentration versus time curves for the same dose given as an intramuscular injection or oral dose (▨) or as a bolus intravenous injection (◪). For these curves the entire dose is absorbed so that the areas under the two curves are the same, For comparison the heavy curve corresponds to absorption of 30% of the dose. The flattening of the concentration curve for oral or i.m. administration minimizes the possibility that the concentration will exceed toxic levels, and it reduces the early elimination of the drug.

For a drug with constant clearance, the availability can be calculated from a comparison of the area under the curve, AUC, following the test dose given by the route under investigation with the area under the curve, AUC_{iv}, following the same size dose given intravenously (see Fig.6.3). After an intravenous dose the entire dose, D, reaches the general circulation and is then eliminated so (see Section 2.1)

$$D = CL \cdot AUC_{iv}$$

Exceptions are drugs metabolized in plasma or the lungs. Following any other dose form, the plasma concentration rises gradually to a maximum then falls as indicated in Fig. 10.2 and the absorbed dose can be calculated as

$$absorbed \ dose = CL \cdot AUC$$

Changing the dosage form shouldn't alter the clearance, so

$$F = \frac{absorbed \ dose}{given \ dose} = \frac{AUC}{AUC_{iv}}$$

6.4   THE AVERAGE RATE OF DRUG ABSORPTION

Over a period of time that is long compared to the interval between doses, the average rate of drug absorption must be

$$R_{av,in} = \frac{\text{amount absorbed}}{\text{elapsed time}}$$

(Mathematically, if the rate of absorption is plotted as a function of time, the average equals the ratio of the area under the curve to the elapsed time. This area also equals the amount absorbed.) **If the same dose, D, is repeated at a regular interval, τ,** then both the amount absorbed and the elapsed time are simply proportional to the number of doses, and

$$R_{av,in} = \frac{D \cdot F}{\tau}$$

Thus **the average rate of absorption and the average concentration at steady state** (see Section 2.1) **depend on the dose rate and the fraction absorbed but not explicitly on the rate of absorption of each dose. Changes in the processes that determine the rate will often affect the average rate, but only because they change the fraction absorbed.**

It may at first be surprising that the average, steady-state rate of absorption does not depend explicitly on the rate at which each dose is absorbed. To understand why, it may help to consider two formulations that are completely absorbed, one very rapidly and the other slowly. For the first, absorption is very fast at the start of a dose interval but almost zero by the end. Furthermore only one dose is being absorbed at a time. Thus for this formulation the average rate of absorption during a dose interval is much less than the high peak rate of absorption for the single dose. By contrast, if absorption of each dose is slow, the peak rate is low but absorption of a dose persists throughout the interval and several following intervals as well. Thus during any interval the average rate of absorption (from all the doses) is much higher than the low peak rate (from a single dose). The earlier argument shows that the two averages, one much less than a high peak and the other much greater than a low peak, are in fact the same.

7 THE STEADY-STATE VOLUME OF DISTRIBUTION

To maintain a steady-state concentration a drug must be administered at the rate that just balances elimination. If dosing is started at this rate, drug will accumulate in the body until the plasma concentration is high enough and elimination fast enough for balance to be achieved. For most drugs the amount that must be accumulated is proportional to the intended average plasma concentration, $C_{av,ss}$. The proportionality constant,

$$V_{ss} = \frac{\text{average amount in the body at steady state}}{C_{av,ss}}$$

is called the steady-state volume of distribution. V_{ss} equals the volume of a well mixed fluid with concentration $C_{av,ss}$, that would contain the average, steady-state amount in the body. Because the volume of distribution increases proportionally with body size it is often stated per unit of body weight. Thus a volume of distribution of 50 litre for a 70 kg man would be 0.71 litre kg^{-1}.

In the steady state the average amount in each tissue is constant and, excepting the sites of absorption and elimination, there is no net movement of the substance between the plasma and the tissues. Therefore, **unless the drug is eliminated at many sites, V_{ss} for a drug depends only on its equilibrium distribution and not on factors like the clearance, blood flows, permeability, etc. This equilibrium distribution is determined by the regions of the body accessible to the drug and its binding**.

The steady-state volume of distribution also relates the average concentration during dosing to the amount that must be eliminated from the body when dosing is stopped. The ability to estimate this amount can be important in the treatment of drug overdose.

7.1 EXPERIMENTAL DETERMINATION OF V_{ss}

At least in principle V_{ss} can be calculated simply from data obtained using an infusion at a constant rate, R_0. The amount present at steady state equals the total amount eliminated after the infusion is stopped. This amount can be measured directly for the few drugs that are eliminated solely by excretion in the urine.

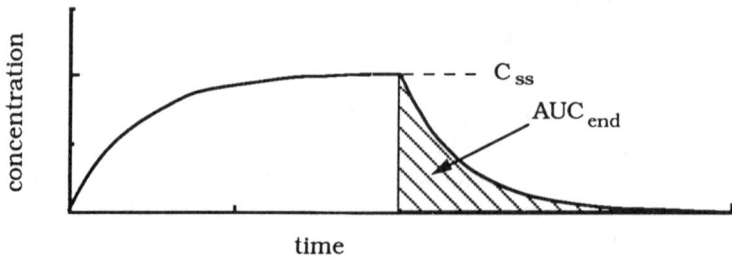

Figure 7.1 The area under the curve AUCafter the end of an infusion. The steady-state volume of distribution can be calculated from this area as described in the text.

It can also be calculated as $CL \cdot AUC_{end}$ if the clearance is a constant. AUC_{end} is defined in Fig. 7.1. Because $CL = R_0/C_{ss}$, the definition of V_{ss} becomes

$$V_{ss} = \frac{CL \cdot AUC_{end}}{C_{ss}} = \frac{R_0 AUC_{end}}{C_{ss}^2}$$

In practice V_{ss} is usually calculated from single-dose data as described in Supplements 3 and 4.

7.2   FACTORS THAT DETERMINE V_{ss}

If a substance can reach more places or more of it is bound in the tissues, then for the same free concentration the total amount in the body will be larger and the volume of distribution will be greater.   The effects of changes in plasma protein-binding are considered in Supplement 2.

The portions of the body which are accessible to a substance depend upon the barriers it can cross. These barriers include the capillary walls, the cell membranes, and the blood-brain barrier.

7.2.1 Peripheral capillary walls

All substances with a radius less than about 3 nm including virtually all drugs are highly permeant across peripheral capillary walls. Lipid-soluble substances go straight through the cells, while polar substances cross through slits between them. Large molecules can also cross peripheral capillary walls, but very much less rapidly. **Even serum albumin is continually leaking out of the capillaries and venules and being returned to**

the blood system via the lymphatics. **All drugs that reach the plasma have access to the peripheral interstitial space.** However, because they may bind to different extents in the plasma and in the interstitial fluid, the total concentrations in plasma and interstitial fluid can be quite different.

7.2.2 Cell membranes

All lipid-soluble molecules smaller than the lipids themselves are able to cross cell membranes. Water, methanol and ethanol are sufficiently lipid-soluble. **Larger or more polar substances like urea, glucose, K^+, etc. need specific transporters.** A few drugs can use such transporters, for instance guanethidine gains access to sympathetic nerve terminals using the transporter for noradrenaline called uptake 1. However, as a rule, if a drug is to reach a target within cells, it must be sufficiently lipid-soluble.

7.2.3 Blood-brain barrier

Capillaries in the central nervous system differ from those in the periphery in that the capillary wall is not freely permeable to small polar substances. Thus **for drugs to gain access to the CNS they must either be lipid-soluble or be transported by the special systems.** An important example of a polar substance that does enter is L-dopa which presumably uses a transporter for amino acids. Dopamine, which is produced from L-dopa by decarboxylation, cannot cross.

Given enough time, with a high plasma concentration appreciable amounts of many substances would be able to cross the blood-brain barrier. However, the cerebrospinal fluid which bathes the brain is not static. It is formed actively with controlled composition in the choroid plexus at about $0.3 \, ml \, min^{-1}$ and removed at the same rate by bulk flow in the arachnoid villi. Since its volume is about 200 ml, 10% is removed per hour. For the drug concentration in the CSF to reach any given concentration it must be infused at a rate that continually replaces the drug that is swept away. Very small leaks across the blood-brain barrier produce negligible concentrations. In effect polar drugs don't reach the brain from plasma.

7.3   VOLUME OF DISTRIBUTION, ANATOMICAL VOLUMES, AND MARKERS

It is important to realize that the steady-state volume of distribution is an equivalent or apparent volume. It can be represented as the volume of a beaker of fluid; only rarely does it correspond to an actual anatomical volume. For example a relatively large amount of a drug like propranolol is bound in the tissues. Its steady-state volume of distribution is about 270 litre or 3.9 litre kg^{-1}, almost four times the entire volume of the body. Because total body water is roughly 42 litre and the total concentration in plasma is always at least as great as the free concentration, **values of V_{ss} much greater than 40-42 litre (0.6 litre kg^{-1}) require that the drug is bound extensively in the tissues or that it is soluble in fat.**

Because the factors which determine binding are so unpredictable, it is difficult to predict the steady-state volume of distribution from the structure and physical properties of a substance. However, there are a few substances whose volumes of distribution are sufficiently easy to interpret that they can be used to measure anatomical volumes.

7.3.1   Plasma volume

If almost all of a substance in the body is bound to plasma proteins, the steady-state volume of distribution is 7-8 litre (ca 0.1 litre kg^{-1}). This volume is more than double the volume of plasma because more than half the plasma proteins are in the interstitial fluid. However, the circulation of plasma proteins from blood to interstitium, to lymphatics, and back to blood is slow. Following injection, almost all of an extensively bound substance remains in the plasma for several hours and the volume of distribution calculated from a plasma concentration measured within this time is a good approximation to the **plasma volume, (ca 3 litre. or 0.04 litre kg^{-1}).** Substances used in this way as markers are the dye Evan's Blue and radiolabelled iodinated serum albumin Almost all of the anticoagulant, warfarin, is bound to plasma proteins and thus it shows the same behaviour.

7.3.2   Extracellular fluid

A drug or marker has a steady-state volume of distribution equal to the volume of the extracellular fluid when (a) the ratio of the bound and free concentrations is either very small everywhere or the same in the interstitial fluid and plasma, (b) the substance can reach all portions of the extracellular fluid, and (c) it cannot cross cell membranes. Markers that have been used to measure the extracellular fluid volume include inulin, sulphate, and the ^{51}Cr-EDTA complex (EDTA is ethylenediaminetetraacetic acid). (For some purposes it is also possible to use ^{24}Na.) Values ranging from **15 to 18 litre (ca 0.25 litre kg^{-1})**, are quoted for this volume, partly because there is some ambiguity as to what should be included (e.g. transcellular fluids like CSF, aqueous humour, and the contents of the gut?), and partly because approximate methods are often used to measure the volume of distribution. Highly polar drugs with little binding that have volumes of distribution in this range include the aminoglycosides and fluorouracil.

7.3.3   Total body water

The volume of distribution of a substance approaches the volume of total body water, **40-42 litre (ca 0.6 litre kg^{-1})** if it has access to all portions of the body and it binds everywhere only to the same extent as water. The preferred marker substance is tritiated water. Exchange of the tritium atoms with hydrogen atoms that are part of proteins, lipids, etc. is a theoretical problem, but in practice the number of such hydrogen atoms that can exchange within a few hours is much smaller than the number of water molecules. A few drugs distribute in this manner: antipyrine (=phenazone), a weak analgesic now sometimes used as a marker in studies of hepatic function, acyclovir, an antiviral agent, and, approximately, ethanol.

PART II
THE TIME COURSE OF
DRUG CONCENTRATIONS

For most drugs the average, steady-state plasma concentration is completely determined by the dose rate, the availability and the clearance. However dosage regimens that produce the same average concentrations can still lead to markedly different clinical effects. Twelve paracetamol tablets may provide relief from a headache for an entire day if two are taken every four hours, but they certainly won't if all twelve are taken at once. Thus it is important to know at least a little about how the plasma concentration changes between doses. Chapters 8 to 11 present simple approximations that are usually adequate to describe these changes. The principles are applied to data for clinically important drugs in the Exercises at the end of the book. Chapter 12 goes beyond the simple approximations to provide a more physiological description of the time course of induction and recovery from anaesthesia.

8 PLASMA CONCENTRATION AFTER AN INTRAVENOUS BOLUS DOSE

The arterial plasma concentration of a drug increases during an intravenous injection, starts to fall rapidly as soon as the injection is complete, and then settles to a more leisurely rate of decline. The distinction between the faster and slower phases can often be seen by inspecting a plot of the logarithm of the concentration versus time (see Fig. 8.1b). Frequently in such a semilogarithmic plot, the later part of the data can be fitted by a straight line.

8.1 THE TERMINAL PHASE

If after some initial period the concentration following an intravenous dose falls exponentially with time, the exponential portion of the time course is called the terminal phase of drug elimination. The exponential relation (Fig. 8.1a),

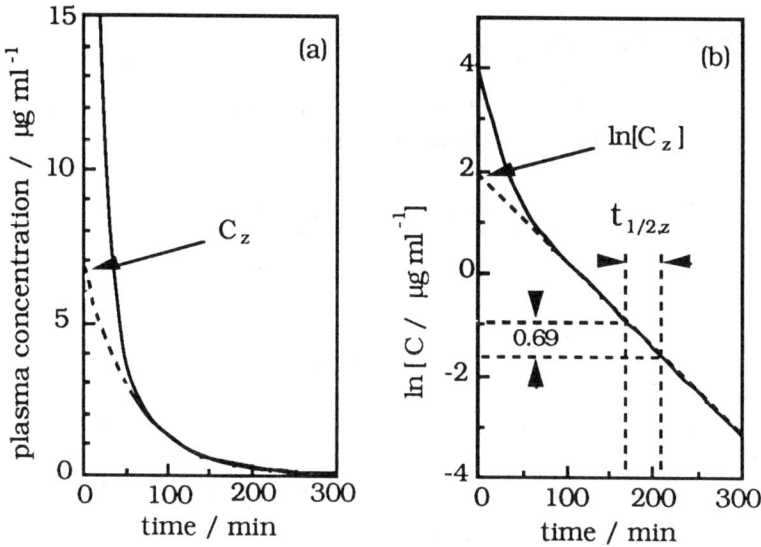

Figure 8.1   Comparison of plots of (a) the concentration versus time and (b) the natural logarithm of the concentration versus time following a 500 mg intravenous dose of oxacillin. In each the upper curve represents the "data" while the lower curve or line is a plot of $C_z e^{-\lambda_z t}$ vs. t. The magnitude of the slope of the straight line on the ln plot, λ_z, is called the terminal phase rate constant for elimination; the intercept on the ln[C] axis is $\ln[C_z]$. The half-life is the time taken for the concentration to fall by half or equivalently for ln[C] to decrease by 0.69. During the terminal phase the half-life is constant. This figure isbased on pharmacokinetic constants (see Table E.4) reported by L.W. Dittert, W.O. Griffen Jr, J.C. LaPiana, F.J. Shainfeld & J.T. Doluisio (1970), *Antimicrobial Agents and Chemotherapy*, **1969**,42-48.

$$C = C_z\, e^{-\lambda_z t}$$

is equivalent to a straight line on a plot of ln[C] versus time (Fig. 8.1b),

$$\ln[C] = \ln[C_z] - \lambda_z t$$

λ_z **is called the terminal phase rate constant for elimination** and C_z is the terminal phase intercept, "z" is used for the subscript as it is the terminal letter of the alphabet. While C_z and λ_z completely describe the terminal phase time course, these values are rarely reported. Instead it is conventional to tabulate the clearance and the half-life.

8.2 THE HALF-LIFE

The half-life is defined as the time taken for the plasma concentration to fall to half its value. To find the half-life in the terminal phase, $t_{1/2,z}$, pick a concentration C_i and locate $\ln[C_i]$ on the line for the terminal phase. The half-life is then the time taken for $\ln[C]$ to decrease from this initial value to $\ln[C_i/2]$, i.e. the time for $\ln[C]$ to decrease by

$$\ln[C_i] - \ln[C_i/2] = \ln[C_i/(C_i/2)] = \ln[2] = 0.69.$$

If we consider instead the fall from $\ln[C_i/2]$ to $\ln[C_i/4]$ then because the plot is a straight line, the time taken to halve the concentration is the same as before. In other words the half-life is a constant throughout the terminal phase. **An exponential fall in concentration is synonymous with a constant half-life.**

The terminal phase half-life, $t_{1/2,z}$ is simply related to the rate constant λ_z. The slope of the line on the plot of $\ln[C]$ versus time is just the ratio of the change in $\ln[C]$ to the change in time,

$$\text{slope} = \frac{\Delta\ln[C]}{\Delta t} = -\lambda_z$$

For $\Delta t = t_{1/2,z}$ the change in $\ln[C]$ is -0.69 so

$$\lambda_z = \frac{0.69}{t_{1/2,z}}$$

The use of semi-log paper to calculate the half-life and rate constant is illustrated in Fig. S3.1 in the Supplementary Topics. Data for practice calculations are provided in Tables E.1-E.3, E.5 and E.6.

For many drugs the terminal phase is reached before most of the drug is eliminated. For these the half-life of clinical interest is $t_{1/2,z}$. For others, e.g. gentamicin and methotrexate, the concentration falls to low values with constant half-life (the value found in tables), but the true terminal phase is much more prolonged (see Section S1.2). For still others with markedly non-linear elimination like ethanol and phenytoin there is no phase with a constant half-life until the concentrations fall to very low values.

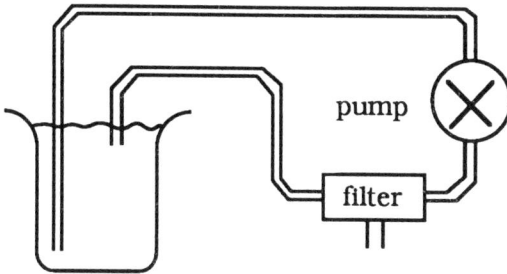

Figure 8.2. A beaker model for the pharmacokinetics of a drug.

8.3 FACTORS THAT DETERMINE THE HALF-LIFE:
THE BODY AS A BEAKER

The conventional approximate approach to predicting changes in plasma concentrations (see Fig. 8.2) is equivalent to a model in which the body is represented by a fluid-filled beaker. A pump mixes the fluid and circulates it past a filter that indicates a route of elimination. The clearance, which is assumed constant, and the volume of fluid are chosen so that the concentration in the beaker, whether in the steady state or following a bolus dose, will be as close as possible to the plasma concentration in the body.

The half-life of the drug in the beaker, $t_{1/2,beaker}$, is determined by the relation between the amount in the beaker and the rate of elimination. This relation depends on the volume, V_{beaker}, and the clearance, CL_{beaker}. By definition during one half-life elimination reduces the concentration from C to C/2. Because the amount in the beaker is simply proportional to the concentration

$$A = V_{beaker}C$$

as the concentration is halved so is the amount present, and the amount eliminated in one half-life equals one half of the amount present at the start. But by the definition of "average" the same amount eliminated is equal to the product of the half-life and the average elimination rate during the half-life. Thus the half-life is

$$t_{1/2,beaker} = \frac{(1/2) \cdot (\text{initial amount})}{(\text{average elimination rate over the half-life})}$$

At the start, when the concentration is C, the elimination rate is $CL_{beaker}C$. At the end, when the concentration is $C/2$, it will be $CL_{beaker}C/2$. A good first guess for the average is half way between these two limits, i.e. $3/4$ of the initial rate (see Fig. 2.1). Using this guess, the half-life is approximately

$$t_{1/2,beaker} = \frac{(1/2) \cdot (\text{initial amount})}{(3/4) \cdot (\text{initial elimination rate})}$$

The constant $2/3 = 0.67$ isn't quite right because the average rate of elimination (equal to $CL \cdot C_{av}$ as in Fig. 2.1) is in fact a little smaller than half way between the extremes (see Supplement 5). The correct constant for an interval equal to one half-life is $\ln[2] = 0.69$ and

$$t_{1/2,beaker} = 0.69 \, \frac{\textbf{initial amount}}{\textbf{initial elimination rate}}$$

Because the initial amount is $V_{beaker}C$ and the initial rate of elimination is $CL_{beaker}C$ this can be rewritten as

$$t_{1/2,beaker} = 0.69 \, \frac{V_{beaker}}{CL_{beaker}}$$

For a beaker with constant clearance the half-life is a constant independent of concentration and time. Thus an exponential fall in plasma concentration is seen because both the rate of elimination and the amount of drug remaining in the beaker are proportional to the plasma concentration and thus to each other. The rate of decrease of the amount present is therefore proportional to the amount present just as for radioactive decay.

The half-life is longer if the volume is larger because more drug must be eliminated to change the amount by half. The half-life is shorter if the clearance is larger because drug is eliminated faster at each concentration.

The pharmacokinetics of the elimination of a drug from a beaker with initial concentration C_0 and constant clearance may be summarized as follows:

$$\text{rate of elimination} = CL_{beaker} \, C = k_{el} \, A$$

$$A = V_{beaker} \, C \qquad k_{el} = CL_{beaker}/V_{beaker}$$

$$C = C_0 e^{-k_{el}t} \quad \text{and} \quad t_{1/2,beaker} = 0.69/k_{el}$$

where k_{el} is the rate constant for elimination from the beaker.

For a beaker with constant clearance the half-life is completely determined by the clearance and the volume. Real people or animals aren't well stirred beakers. The extent to which such a simple model can be used to describe the body is pursued in the following sections.

8.4   THE REAL VARIATION OF PLASMA CONCENTRATION WITH TIME

Drugs are taken to and removed from each tissue by the blood. When a "typical" drug is first injected the proportions delivered to different destinations within the body are determined by the relative blood flows. During the injection and for the next minute or so most of the drug enters the tissues with particularly high blood flow (including the plasma), some is taken to sites of elimination, and the rest goes to other tissues. For technical reasons this very early part of the distribution of a drug has rarely been measured. The distribution at this stage is indicated in Fig. 8.3.

During the next, "initial" phase the plasma concentration decreases both because drug is eliminated and because the drug continues to diffuse out of the plasma in the low blood flow tissues. As a result of the combination of elimination and distribution the fractional decrease per unit time is relatively large and on the log plot (Fig. 8.1b) the curve is steep. For many drugs this phase lasts for 20 to 60 min. The initial phase for thiopentone is discussed in Chapter 12.

Later, during the terminal phase (see Fig. 8.4), drug is still removed from the blood that goes to the sites of elimination, but it is added back to the plasma that flows through all other tissues. Now, because these additions and removals partially cancel, the fractional change in plasma concentration per unit time is smaller and the curve on the log plot is less steep. During the terminal phase the drug concentrations decrease together in all parts of the body.

The drug concentration in a well stirred beaker of fluid cannot possibly be the same as the plasma concentration at all times after a dose. In a beaker the drug is immediately spread over all the volume. In the body at the time of injection the drug appears to be present in only the plasma and those parts of high blood flow tissues that can be penetrated rapidly. Thus at this

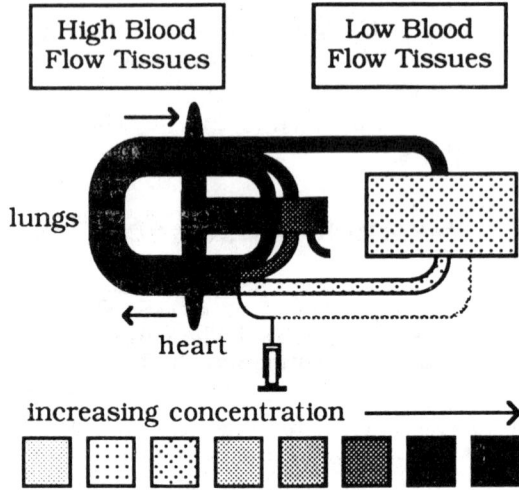

Figure 8.3 A simplified model for the distribution of a drug in the body (see also Fig's. 8.4 and 8.5) showing the distribution of a drug a minute or two after the end of an intravenous bolus dose, i.e. at the start of the initial phase of drug elimination. The tissues of the body are represented by two groups, those with high blood flow and those with low blood flow per unit weight. The size of the blood vessels supplying each group is roughly proportional to the fraction of cardiac output going to all the tissues of that type. High blood flow tissues include the brain, heart, lungs, liver, and kidneys. Low blood flow tissues include muscle and skin. More realistic models for the body would divide each tissue into extracellular and intracellular components. Elimination is represented as the small pipe emerging from the part of the high blood flow tissues with a somewhat lower concentration. The shading of each tissue indicates the concentration in plasma that would be at equilibrium with the amount of drug present in the tissue. For the "typical" drug of this figure, at the start of the initial phase the concentration in high blood flow tissues is close to that in plasma. By contrast the concentration in low blood flow tissues is still low because in the short period of the injection each element of tissue has had delivered to it only a small amount of drug. In effect the drug appears to be distributed over only part of the body.

time the volume of a model beaker would be relatively small and the apparent half-life is short. Subsequently, as the drug is distributed to the rest of the body, the size of the corresponding beaker and the half-life increase to their terminal values. These statements can be made quantitative in terms of the volume of distribution.

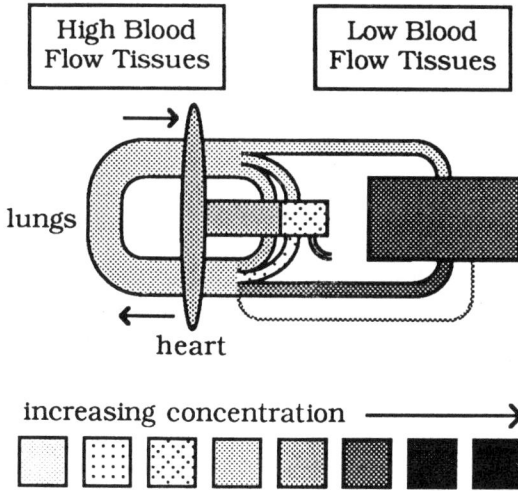

Figure 8.4 The distribution of a drug during the terminal phase. (See the legend to Fig. 8.3 for explanation of the symbols.) During the terminal phase elimination reduces the concentration in the plasma emerging from the liver and/or the kidneys. This reduces the concentration in the plasma of mixed venous blood and arterial plasma so that it is lower than would be at equilibrium with the tissues. Drug is thus returned to plasma from both high and low blood flow tissues and taken to the sites of elimination.

8.5 THE VOLUME OF DISTRIBUTION

The volume of distribution of a substance, defined as the ratio

$$V_d = \frac{\text{amount in body}}{\text{arterial plasma concentration}} = \frac{A}{C}$$

is not a constant. It can have very different values depending upon the circumstances. The most important of these values, the steady-state volume of distribution, was considered in the previous chapter.

8.5.1 The initial volume of distribution

If the drug has just been given intravenously, a large fraction of the amount within the body is in the plasma or in organs with high blood flow (see Fig. 8.3). The arterial plasma concentration is therefore relatively high, and the initial value of the volume of distribution, $V_{initial}$, is low. An approximate value of $V_{initial}$ can be estimated from experimental records as dose divided by the concentration obtained by extrapolating a curve fitted to the measured concentrations back to the time of the injection. Typical values range from plasma volume, 3 litres, up to 30 litres. Values for $V_{initial}$ are rarely if ever needed in clinical applications (see Section 9.2).

8.5.2   The terminal phase volume of distribution

During a terminal phase, the half-life is constant and the plasma concentration falls exponentially as if the body were a beaker containing drug at the same concentration as in plasma. So that the concentration in the body and the concentration in the beaker will be equal throughout the terminal phase, the rate constant for elimination from the beaker, $k_{el} = CL_{beaker}/V_{beaker}$, must be equal to the terminal phase rate constant, λ_z. Furthermore, for the rates of elimination from the body and the beaker to be equal, the clearances must be the same. **The volume of this beaker can then be calculated from the rate constant λ_z and clearance CL as** (see Section 8.3)

$$V_z = \frac{\alpha}{\lambda_z} = \frac{\alpha \cdot t_{1/2,z}}{0.69}$$

This terminal phase volume of distribution, V_z, is in fact the actual volume of distribution (defined as A/C) for the drug in the terminal phase. Because elimination from the beaker and the body occur at the same rate, $CL \cdot C$, the same total amount is eliminated from each during the terminal phase, i.e. they both contain the same amount of drug and the ratios of amount to concentration are also the same.

V_z is often called V_{area} because it is usually calculated from a measurement of the area under the curve. Recall that the clearance may be calculated from the area under the curve after a single dose as,

$$CL = \frac{\text{absorbed dose}}{AUC}$$

and thus

$$V_z = V_{area} = \frac{\text{absorbed dose}}{\lambda_z AUC}$$

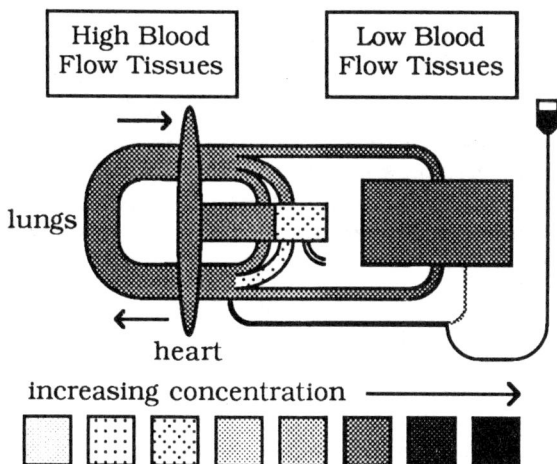

Figure 8.5 The distribution of a drug in the body at steady state. (See the legend to Fig. 8.3 for explanation of the symbols.) The drug is continuously being infused into a peripheral vein and eliminated in the liver or the kidneys such that the amount taken out of plasma by the elimination is just replaced by the infusion. The amount in most tissues is at equilibrium with the concentration in arterial plasma.

8.5.3 The relation between V_z and V_{ss}

In the steady state the amount of drug in most tissues is at equilibrium with the concentration in arterial plasma (see Fig. 8.5). If the body were a beaker, this equilibrium would hold at all times and the volume of distribution in the terminal phase, V_z, would be the same as the steady-state volume of distribution, V_{ss}. However, **in the terminal phase** there must be diffusion of drug from the tissues back into the plasma as this is how the drug is removed and taken to the sites of elimination. Thus there must be a gradient of free drug concentration between the tissues and plasma because it is this gradient which drives the diffusion. But if the free concentration in the tissues is greater than C, then **the amount of drug in the tissues is greater than would be at equilibrium with the plasma concentration** and

$$V_z = \frac{\text{terminal phase amount}}{C} > \frac{\text{equilibrium amount}}{C} = V_{ss}$$

that is

$$V_z > V_{ss}$$

Unlike the steady-state volume of distribution, V_z changes whenever the clearance changes. If drug is eliminated rapidly from the plasma compared to the rate at which it can get out of the tissues, then the plasma concentration falls below equilibrium with the tissues, and the ratio of amount to plasma concentration is relatively large, i.e. V_z is clearly greater than V_{ss}. In practical terms, **when diffusion of a drug from the tissues to plasma is a relatively slow process compared to elimination from plasma, the terminal half-life is substantially longer than would be predicted from the clearance and the steady-state volume of distribution, so that**

$$t_{1/2,z} = \frac{0.69 \cdot V_z}{CL} > \frac{0.69 \cdot V_{ss}}{CL}$$

For instance, for the data displayed in Fig 8.1, $V_z = 29$ litre, $V_{ss} = 16$ litre, and the half-life is 50 min instead of 30 min (see also Sections E.2.3 and E.2.10). By contrast, if the drug is eliminated relatively slowly, then the concentration in plasma will be near to equilibrium with the tissues and the steady-state and terminal phase volumes of distribution will be similar, $V_z = V_{ss}$. Drug distribution and changes in the volume of distribution are considered in more detail in Supplement 1.

8.6   THE SINGLE COMPARTMENT MODEL

Whenever a plot of ln[C] vs t is a single straight line with slope λ_z, the plasma concentration behaves as if the body were a single compartment or beaker. The area under the curve can then be found using calculus as

$$AUC_z = \int_0^\infty Cdt = \int_0^\infty C_0 e^{-\lambda_z t} dt = \frac{C_z}{\lambda_z} = \frac{C_z t_{1/2,z}}{0.69}$$

The clearance from the single compartment, CL_{sc}, is then

$$CL_{sc} = \frac{D}{AUC_z} = \frac{D \lambda_z}{C_z} = \frac{0.69D}{C_z t_{1/2,z}}$$

and the only available estimate of the volume of distribution is

$$V_{sc} = \frac{CL_{sc}}{\lambda_z} = \frac{D}{C_z}$$

If a single exponential fits the data accurately, then

$$V_{ss} = V_z = V_{sc}$$

Because the half-life, $t_{1/2,z}$, and the initial concentration, C_z, are so easily determined (see Fig. 8.1 and Section S4.1), **the assumption that the body is a single-compartment** (i.e. it acts like a beaker at all times) **is often used as an approximation** even when a single exponential doesn't fit the data. The approximation then introduces errors into the constants. The total amounts eliminated from the single-compartment beaker and the actual body must both equal the dose. Because the elimination in any short period of time is the product of the clearance and the concentration and the concentrations in the single-compartment beaker are sometimes less and never greater than in the actual body (see the solid and dashed curves in Fig. 8.1), the single-compartment clearance must be greater than the actual clearance. Quantitatively because the amount eliminated equals the product of the clearance and the area under the curve,

$$D = CL_{sc}AUC_z = CL \cdot AUC$$

and thus

$$\frac{CL_{sc}}{CL} = \frac{AUC}{AUC_z}$$

It also follows that during the terminal phase the single-compartment model predicts a rate of elimination that is larger than the actual rate because it uses the correct concentrations but a clearance that is too large. Therefore during the terminal phase a greater amount is eliminated from the beaker than the actual body. But that means during the terminal phase the beaker of the single-compartment model must contain more drug to be eliminated than the actual body even though the concentrations are the same, i.e. $V_{sc} > V_z$. Because the rate constant for elimination is the same in the model and in the body,

$$\frac{V_{sc}}{V_z} = \frac{CL_{sc}}{CL}.$$

There is less elimination from the single-compartment beaker than from the actual body during the initial phase.

The single-compartment model can provide useful quick estimates of the clearance and the volume of distribution from data obtained after an intravenous bolus dose (see Section E.1.1). **However, for dose calculations it is much better to use the correct clearance which can be calculated directly from the data using the area under the curve.**

9 INTRAVENOUS INFUSION

Intravenous infusions are used to obtain a rapid rise in plasma concentration or to insure accurate control. The net rate at which drug accumulates in the body during an infusion (see Fig. 9.1) is the difference between the rates of infusion, R_0, and elimination, $CL \cdot C$. As the concentration increases, the rate of elimination increases while the rate of accumulation and the rate of increase in concentration both decrease towards zero. In the steady state the rates of infusion and elimination are equal and the plateau or steady-state concentration, C_{ss}, is related to the clearance by

$$C_{ss} = \frac{R_0}{CL} = \frac{K_o}{Clp.}$$

When the infusion is stopped, elimination decreases the amount in the body, initially at a rate $CL\,C_{ss}$. As the concentration falls, the elimination rate also falls and the concentration decreases less rapidly. Eventually the concentration, the rate of elimination and the rate of change of the concentration all approach zero.

The amount that must be accumulated in the approach to the steady state is the same as the amount that must be eliminated when the infusion is stopped. Furthermore the initial rate at

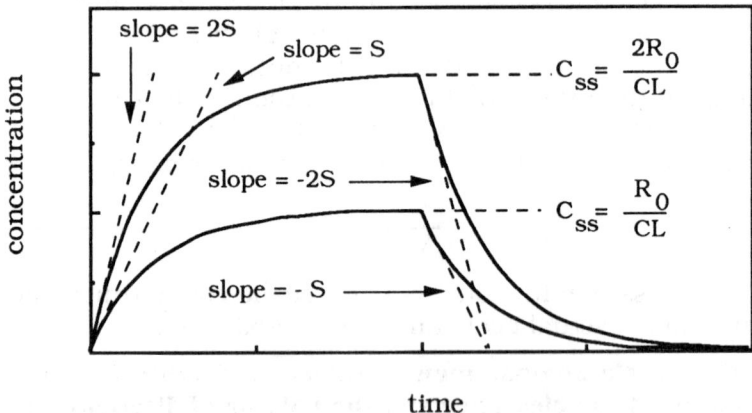

Figure 9.1 Concentrations during and after infusions at rates R_0 and $2R_0$. Both the initial slopes of the curves and the steady-state or plateau concentrations, C_{ss}, are proportional to the infusion rate. The rate of infusion has no effect on the time taken for the concentration, C, to reach any fraction of C_{ss}.

which drug accumulates in the body at the start is the same as the
initial rate of elimination at the end, i.e. $R_0 = CL \cdot C_{ss}$. For drugs
whose concentrations after a single dose are proportional to the
size of the dose, the changes at the beginning and end of a long
infusion are mirror images.

9.1   INFUSION INTO A BEAKER

It is customary when describing the plasma concentration during
a constant infusion to treat the body as if it were a beaker (see
Section S4.3 in the Supplements). Even when this approximation
is poor, so long as the correct value of the clearance is used, the
most important property of the time course, the steady-state
concentration, will be correct.

9.11 The end of an infusion

At the end of an infusion just as after a single intravenous dose
the rate of elimination is equal to the product $CL \cdot C$,

$$\text{the amount in the body} = \frac{\text{the amount still to}}{\text{be eliminated}} = V_{beaker}\, C,$$

and the concentration decreases exponentially with time from
the initial value, C_{ss}, to the final value, 0,

$$C = C_{ss}\, e^{-k_{el}t}$$

So that the second important property of the time course of the
concentration, the half-life, will also be correct, the rate constant
for elimination from the beaker, $k_{el} = CL/V_{beaker}$, should be equal
to the terminal phase rate constant, $\lambda_z = CL/V_z$, i.e. $V_{beaker} = V_z$ and

$$C = C_{ss}\, e^{-\lambda_z t}$$

9.1.2   The start of an infusion

**At the start of the infusion the total change in concentration is
the same as at the end, but at the start it is the difference in
concentrations, $C_{ss} - C$, rather than C which is initially equal to
C_{ss} and finally equal to 0.** During the approach to the steady
state,

rate of accumulation = rate of infusion - rate of elimination
$$= R_0 - CL \cdot C = CL \cdot (C_{ss} - C)$$

and

the amount still to be accumulated $= V_z \cdot (C_{ss}-C)$

Thus C_{ss} - C at the start and C at the end have the same initial and final values and change at the same rates. They are, in fact, identical and

$$C_{ss} - C = C_{ss}\, e^{-\lambda_z t}$$

(You may find it helpful to repeat the arguments in Section 8.3, using the amount accumulated in a half-life, $V_z \cdot [C_{ss}-C]/2$, and the average rate of accumulation during the half-life, approximately $3 \cdot CL \cdot [C_{ss}-C]/4$.) More generally, if after reaching an initial steady-state concentration, $C_{initial}$, the infusion rate is changed the concentration approaches the new steady-state concentration, C_{ss}, following

$$C_{ss} - C = (C_{ss} - C_{initial})\, e^{-\lambda_z t}.$$

The half-life, $t_{1/2,z} = 0.69/\lambda_z$, is the same for any change caused by an increase or a decrease in the rate of infusion.

9.1.3   The time taken to reach a concentration

If an infusion is started at the maintenance rate, $CL \cdot C_{ss}$, the time taken to reach any fraction of the final concentration, $1 - C/C_{ss}$, can be estimated by rewriting the exponential relation for infusion into a beaker as

$$t = - \frac{1}{\lambda_z} \ln\left[1 - \frac{C}{C_{ss}}\right]$$

The time to reach any fraction of the final value **increases as the fraction approaches one, is longer for drugs with longer half-lives, but is the same for all rates of infusion. It takes n half-lives for $1 - C/C_{ss}$, to reach $(1/2)^n$.** For a drug like lignocaine (see Fig. 9.2) whose half-life is about 110 min, it will take 110 min to to get to within one half of the final concentration, 220 min to reach within one quarter, 330 min to reach within one eighth, etc. This slow increase in concentration produces complications for two reasons. Firstly, when a lignocaine infusion is started, its antidysrhythmic effects are required within a few minutes, not a few hours. Secondly, it will take a long time to ascertain the steady-state consequences of any infusion rate.

9.2   LOADING DOSES AND PRIMING INFUSIONS

In practice loading doses are required whenever it is important to reach effective concentrations in less than a half-life. Loading doses can be administered by giving an additional series of injections or by infusing at higher rates until the desired concentration is reached. **The amount of drug which must be loaded to reach the steady-state is $C_{ss}V_{ss}$** (i.e. it is the amount which would be required to produce the desired concentration in a beaker of volume V_{ss}). **However,** when first injected most of the drug is either in the plasma or in tissues with high blood flow such as the heart, liver, kidneys, and brain (i.e. the drug appears to have been added to a smaller beaker). If it is necessary **to avoid greatly exceeding the maintenance plasma concentration, the amount that can be injected intravenously at any one time is roughly $C_{ss}V_{initial}$ which is usually much less than $C_{ss}V_{ss}$.** For example with lignocaine and $C_{ss} = 2.65\,\mu g\,ml^{-1}$ these amounts are approximately 100 mg and 200 mg respectively (see Fig. 9.2). **Even the reduced amount must be injected slowly to avoid high, potentially toxic plasma concentrations during the injection.**

The dose is first diluted by the blood flowing through the vein at the site of injection and then by the blood it encounters during passage through the heart and lungs (see Fig. 8.3). As a rough approximation the concentration in arterial plasma during the injection can be estimated as the rate of injection divided by the flow of plasma through the chambers of the heart. Thus even a cautious injection of a 100 mg loading dose of lignocaine over 2 min yielding a rate of $50\,mg\,min^{-1}$ would produce arterial plasma entering the blood vessels of the heart and brain with a concentration approaching $50\,mg\,min^{-1} / 3000\,ml\,min^{-1} = 15\,\mu g\,ml^{-1}$ which is about five times higher than the target concentration. The rest of the loading dose can, if necessary, be administered later as one or more injections or as a priming infusion over a period comparable to the duration of the initial phase for the drug. An example calculated from pharmacokinetic constants for lignocaine is shown in Figure 9.2. As noted earlier if only the maintenance infusion is given, hours are required to reach effective concentrations. The addition of a single bolus loading dose, $C_{ss}V_{initial}$, greatly improves matters. There are a number of recipes which combine this bolus dose with a sequence of extra infusions to complete the loading. The failure of the simple beaker model to provide adequate predictions for lignocaine is explored in Section E.2.3.

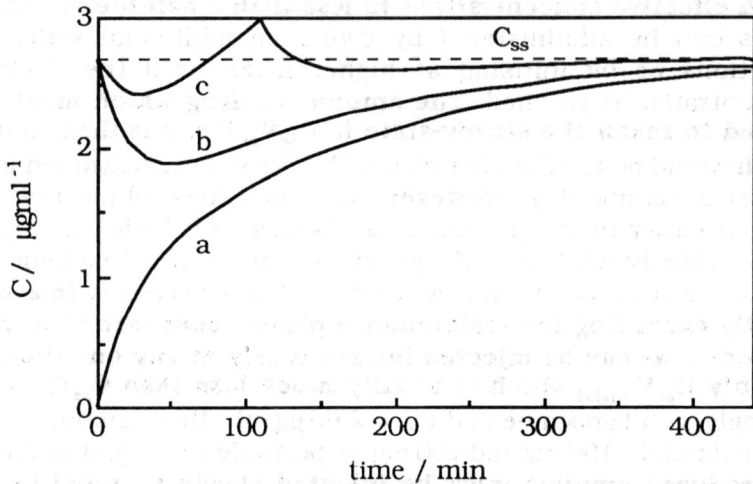

Figure 9.2 Calculated concentrations for lignocaine with a maintenance infusion (a) alone, (b) plus a bolus dose equal to $C_{ss}V_{initial}$, and (c) plus the same bolus dose and a priming infusion at 1.5 times the maintenance rate. The curves have been calculated using CL = 650 ml min⁻¹, V_{ss} = 77 litres, V_z= 103 litres, $V_{initial}$ = 35 litres, and λ_z = 0.0063 min⁻¹ (see Sections E.2.3 and S4.3). After the initial loading dose in (b) and (c) the concentration of lignocaine falls because the rate of infusion is less than the sum of the rate at which lignocaine is being eliminated and the rate at which it is diffusing from the plasma into the tissues. At steady state the rate of infusion must balance only the rate of elimination. The acceptable variation in concentration for lignocaine is controversial. A fall from 2.65 µgml⁻¹ to 1.8 µgml⁻¹ may have clinical consequences. The priming infusion in (c) must be stopped at the right time to avoid toxic concentrations.

10 SIMULTANEOUS ABSORPTION AND ELIMINATION OF A SINGLE DOSE

The time course of absorption varies with the physical properties of the drug, its formulation and the route of administration. After intramuscular injection if the drug remains in solution the rate of absorption will be proportional to the concentration of the drug at the site of the injection and hence to the amount remaining to be absorbed. Alternatively if the drug precipitates, absorption occurs at a nearly constant rate until the solid is exhausted. With oral administration, there is normally a delay in the appearance of drug in the circulation while the tablet disintegrates or until the drug reaches the intestines. Subsequently absorption is proportional to the amount remaining.

When the rate of absorption from a site, R_{in}, is proportional to the amount of the dose remaining, the rate of absorption decreases exponentially with time (compare Section 8.3),

$$R_{in} = k_{in} F \cdot D \cdot e^{-k_{in}t}$$

with a half-life

$$t_{1/2,in} = \frac{0.69}{k_{in}}$$

When the availability, F, of a dose, D, is less than 1, the absorption process is usually assumed to be equivalent to the total absorption of a smaller dose FD.

Normally the absorption half-life is shorter than the elimination half-life (see Fig. 10.1a). Initially, as the drug is absorbed, the amount within the body, the plasma concentration and the rate of elimination all increase while the amount remaining to be absorbed and the rate of absorption both decrease. The maximum concentration occurs when absorption has become slow enough and elimination fast enough for them just to balance. Shortly thereafter absorption is effectively complete and the amount in the body and the plasma concentration decrease as governed by the elimination. The time course of the increase is governed primarily by the half-life for absorption, while the final half-life for the decrease is the half-life for elimination. Rapid absorption is important when effects are required quickly, e.g. for pain relief after taking an aspirin. The factors that affect the rate of absorption are discussed in Chapter 6.

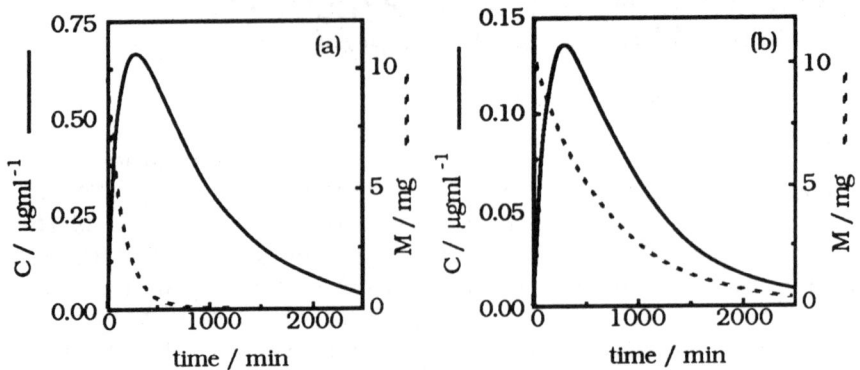

Figure 10.1   The plasma concentration, C, and the amount remaining to be absorbed, M. The rate of absorption, R_{in} equals the rate constant for absorption, k_{in}, times the amount remaining to be absorbed and the rate of elimination equals the clearance times the plasma concentration. In (a) the half-time for absorption is short compared to the half-life for elimination. Shortly after the maximum concentration is reached there is little more absorption and the concentration falls as governed by elimination. The figure is drawn with $t_{1/2,z}$ = 500 min   (λ_z = 0.0069 min^{-1}), $t_{1/2,in}$ = 100 min (k_{in} = 0.0014 min^{-1}), and V_z=10 litre. In part (b) the half-life for absorption is long compared to the half-life for elimination. After the peak, the plasma concentration is close to $C = R_{in}/CL$. The figure is drawn with $t_{1/2,z}$ = 100 min, $t_{1/2,in}$ = 500 min, and V_z=10 litre. Note the difference in the scales for the concentrations in the two parts which corresponds to the five-fold greater clearance in part (b). The effects of changes in k_{in} with constant clearance are shown in Fig. 10.2.

If the absorption half-life is much longer than the elimination half-life (see Fig. 10.1b), the increase in drug concentration occurs while there is little change in the rate of absorption. Thus, just as for an infusion (see Chapter 9), the half-life for the increase in concentration is then the half-life for elimination. Subsequently the rate of the apparent infusion produced by absorption and the (pseudo) steady-state concentration both decrease slowly, and the half-life for the decrease in plasma concentration is the absorption half-life.

Prolonged absorption is the objective of using sustained release preparations for either injections (see Sections 6.1.2 and E.2.9) **or oral doses. For the latter, the usual intention is to maintain plasma concentrations for 12 hours after a single dose so that the drug can be taken twice daily.** Because the total dose administered is much greater than the amount that is intended to be in the body at one time, the timing of the release must be sufficiently reliable to insure that the whole dose can't be absorbed at once. The maximum duration of the sustained release for an oral preparation is limited by the passage time of the dose through the gut into the faeces.

For the same drug, and hence the same rate constant for elimination, **different formulations can lead to different rates of absorption and hence to different time courses for the plasma concentration**. These time courses can be described in relatively simple mathematical terms if the body is treated as a beaker (see Section 8.2) and absorption decreases exponentially with time. The rate of change of the amount in the body equals the difference between the rates of absorption and elimination, i.e.

$$\text{rate of change of } A = k_{in} F \cdot D \cdot e^{-k_{in}t} - k_{el} A$$

The solution of this equation with the "boundary conditions" that the amount is zero both before the dose and a long time after is

$$A = V_{beaker} C = F \cdot D \cdot k_{in} [e^{-k_{el}t} - e^{-k_{in}t}] / [k_{in} - k_{el}]$$

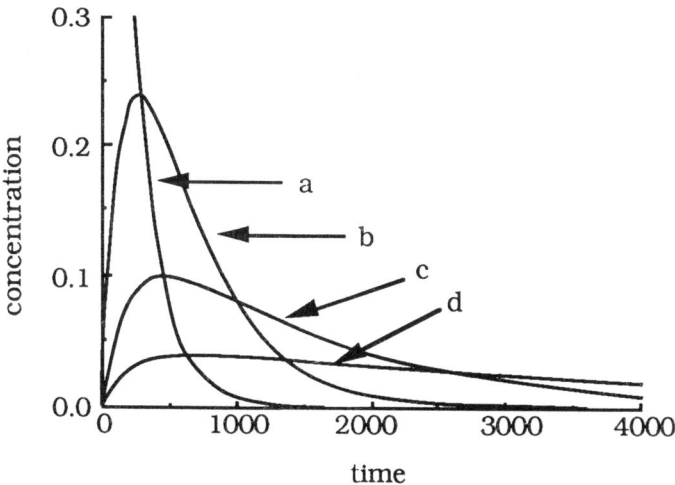

Figure 10.2 The variation in plasma concentration as the formulation is altered to change the rate constant of absorption. The clearance, the fraction absorbed, the area under the curve, the volume of distribution (V_z) and the elimination rate constant ($=0.005\text{min}^{-1}$) are all presumed to remain constant. The rate constant for absorption takes on the following values in min^{-1}: curve a, 0.069; curve b, 0.0023; curve c, 0.00069; and curve d, 0.00023.

11 MULTIPLE DOSES

The toxic effects of a drug limit the maximum dose that can be given and it is rarely practical to achieve a sufficient duration of effect just by increasing the size of the dose. Truly massive doses would be required, e.g. to prolong effects by 10 half-lives would require a 1000 fold increase. Instead of using such large doses, a dose is repeated at intervals, e.g. the 10 extra half-lives might be obtained by repeating the dose once each half-life. For drugs whose concentrations following a dose are proportional to the size of the dose, **the concentrations following multiple doses can be calculated by addition as indicated in Fig. 11.1. All the information needed is available from the response to a single dose and the times of the doses.** Exceptions include drugs with non-linear elimination, e.g. phenytoin, and drugs that induce their own metabolism, e.g. phenobarbitone.

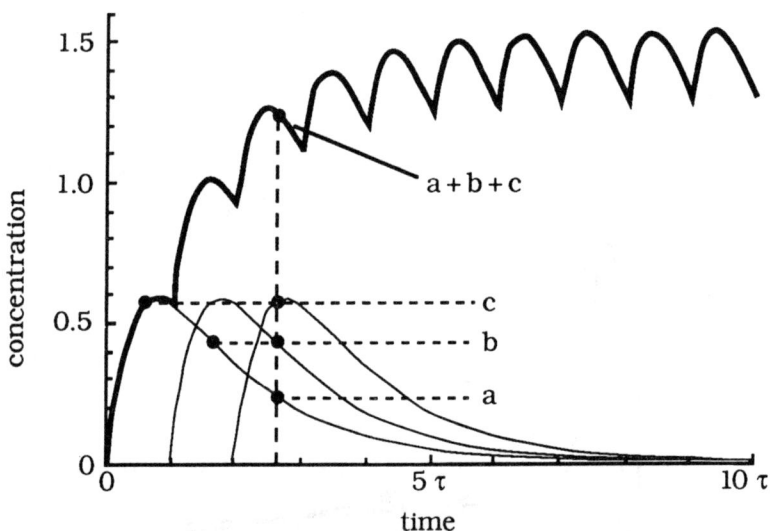

Figure 11.1. The concentrations produced by repetitive administration of a dose with dose interval τ (heavy curve) compared with the concentrations produced by each of the first three doses at times 0, τ, and 2τ (light curves). At any particular time, t_a, the concentration during the series is the sum of the concentrations resulting from all the preceding doses. For instance during the third interval the concentration after the three doses together, a+b+c, is obtained by adding the concentrations a,b, and c. This additivity is sometimes called the Principle of Superposition. Note that a,b, and c can all be read from the response to the first dose as $C(t_a)$, $C(t_a-\tau)$, and $C(t_a-2\tau)$.

11.1 THE AVERAGE STEADY-STATE CONCENTRATION PRODUCED BY REGULAR REPETITION OF A DOSE

In the steady state the average rate of drug absorption must equal the average rate of elimination, i.e. when a dose D is repeated at a regular interval τ (see Sections 2.1 and 6.4), $R_{av,in} = D \cdot F/\tau = CL \cdot C_{av,ss}$. Thus the dose rate, DR, required to maintain an average concentration $C_{av,ss}$ can be calculated from the clearance and the availability as

$$DR = \frac{D}{\tau} = \frac{CL}{F} C_{av,ss}$$

CL/F can be calculated from tabulated values, e.g. those in Goodman & Gilman. Alternatively, **if the response to a single dose of the intended size is known** (see Fig. 11.2), CL/F = D/AUC (see section 6.3) and

$$C_{av,ss} = \frac{AUC}{\tau}$$

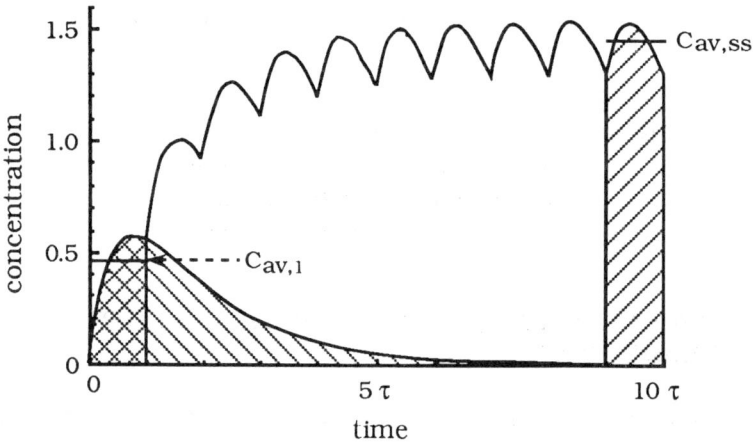

Figure 11.2 The relation between the area under the curve for a single dose, AUC, shown partly as ▨ and partly as ▧, and the area under the curve for the steady state of regular repetition of the same dose, AUC_{ss}, shown as ▨. Because in the steady state the amount absorbed and eliminated in a dose interval, $CL \cdot AUC_{ss}$, must be equal to amount absorbed and eliminated from a single dose, $CL \cdot AUC$, the two areas are equal. $C_{av,ss}$ is the average concentration at steady-state. $C_{av,1}$ is the average concentration and AUC_1, shown as ▨, is the area under the curve for the first dose interval.

11.2   ACCUMULATION RATIO

When multiple doses are given drug accumulates until the plasma concentration is large enough for elimination to balance absorption. **Accumulation from one dose to the next is significant when the next dose is given before most of the previous dose has been eliminated.** This statement is made quantitative by defining the accumulation ratio, AR, as the ratio of the average concentration at steady state to the average concentration during the first dose interval,

$$AR = \frac{C_{av,ss}}{C_{av,1}}$$

Using the definitions of the averages in terms of area under the curve (see Fig. 11.2),

$$AR = \frac{AUC}{\tau} \bigg/ \frac{AUC_1}{\tau}$$

To convert the areas to amounts multiply the top and bottom of this expression by the clearance,

$$AR = \frac{CL \cdot AUC_{ss}}{CL \cdot AUC_1} = \frac{\text{total amount absorbed from one dose}}{\text{amount eliminated in first dose interval}}$$

$$AR = \frac{1}{\left\{ \begin{array}{c} \textbf{the fraction of an absorbed} \\ \textbf{dose that is eliminated} \\ \textbf{in the first dose interval} \end{array} \right\}}$$

11.3 CONCENTRATIONS, DOSE INTERVAL, AND DOSE AT STEADY-STATE

For doses of arbitrary form the variation in concentration between doses is easiest to evaluate graphically or numerically as in Fig. 11.1. However, if absorption of the doses and distribution around the body are both rapid, the maximum and minimum concentrations can be calculated using a beaker model as in Fig. 11.3. These calculations can be turned around to yield estimates for the maximum dose interval,

$$\tau_{max} = \frac{1}{\lambda_z} \ln\frac{C_{max}}{C_{min}} = \frac{t_{1/2 \cdot z}}{0.69} \ln\frac{C_{max}}{C_{min}} = \frac{t_{1/2 \cdot z}}{0.3} \log\frac{C_{max}}{C_{min}}$$

and the maximum dose,

$$D_{max} = \frac{(C_{max} - C_{min}) V_z}{F}$$

consistent with stated maximum and minimum concentrations. Frequently the dose and dose interval are chosen to have convenient values well within these calculated limits. Doses are usually restricted to standard sizes, and dose intervals must fit a daily routine so that they are easy to remember.

11.4   THE TIME TO REACH EFFECTIVE CONCENTRATIONS

If the dose interval is much greater than the half-life for a single dose, then each dose can be considered in isolation and effective concentrations will be reached only if these are achieved by a single dose. **If the dose interval is much less than a half-life,** then multiple dosing is almost the same as an infusion at a rate $R_0 = D$ F/τ and **the time to reach an effective concentration is calculated in just the same manner as for an infusion using**

$$C_{av,ss} - C = C_{av,ss} \, e^{-\lambda_z t}$$

When the dose interval is comparable to the half-life, the time to first reach an effective concentration can be calculated by adding up the effects of successive doses as in Fig. 11.1 or 11.3.

11.5   LOADING DOSE

Some form of loading dose or doses is required whenever it is important to reach effective concentrations in less than a half-life. The total amount that must be loaded to produce the target average concentration in the first dose interval is called the loading dose. Normally this dose will be divided into two or more parts to avoid high peak concentrations and so that the effects of each can be noted before the rest are given.

If administration were started with a maintenance dose, the average concentration over the first dose interval would be $C_{av,1}$. The loading dose is intended to produce $C_{av,ss}$. Thus **provided the average concentration produced is proportional to the dose,**

$$\frac{C_{av,ss}}{\text{loading dose}} = \frac{C_{av,1}}{\text{maintenance dose}}$$

and

$$\textbf{loading dose} = \textbf{AR} \cdot \textbf{D.}$$

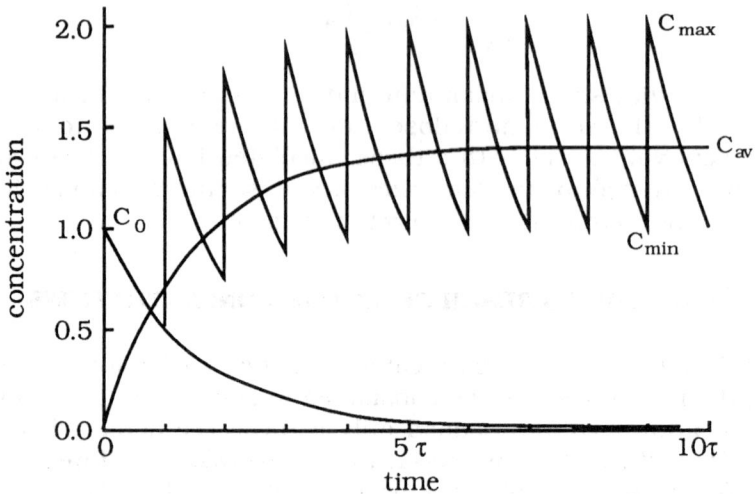

Figure 11.3 The relation between the single-dose and repeated dose concentrations in a beaker model with rapid absorption. So that the model will predict the actual values of the average, steady-state concentration and the terminal phase half-life, its rate constant for elimination must equal λ_z and it must use the actual clearance. The volume of the beaker is then $V_z = CL/\lambda_z$. After each dose at steady-state the concentration falls exponentially

$$C = C_{max} e^{-\lambda_z t}$$

from C_{max} to

$$C_{min} = C_{max} e^{-\lambda_z \tau}.$$

where τ is the dose interval. The next dose then increases the concentration back to C_{max}, i.e.

$$C_{max} = C_0 + C_{min}$$

where C_0 is the concentration produced by a single dose,

$$C_0 = \frac{D \cdot F}{V_z}$$

Combining these relations

$$C_{max} = \frac{D \cdot F}{V_z} \frac{1}{1 - e^{-\lambda_z \tau}} .$$

The accumulation ratio is then

$$AR = \frac{C_{av,ss}}{C_{av,1}} = \frac{C_{max}}{C_0} = \frac{1}{1 - e^{-\lambda_z \tau}}$$

12 ANAESTHETICS

The approximations used in Chapters 8 to 11 are not well suited to describing the distribution of a drug within the body. This chapter introduces physiologically based models, which are, and discusses their application to the use of anaesthetics.

12.1 THIOPENTONE

Thiopentone injected intravenously is widely employed as one of the safest and most convenient agents for the induction of general anaesthesia. If used correctly its effects are very short-lived as a consequence of redistribution between tissues within the body.

Thiopentone crosses cell membranes and the blood-brain barrier rapidly. Thus the concentration in the brain closely follows that in the arterial blood, and **the time between the initial injection and loss of consciousness is only slightly longer than the time taken for the blood carrying the thiopentone to reach the brain. Consciousness is regained when the concentrations in the blood, C_b, and in the brain fall to sufficiently low levels.** The concentration time curve measured in human volunteers (see Fig. 12.1a) has two important features: a fast redistribution (0 to

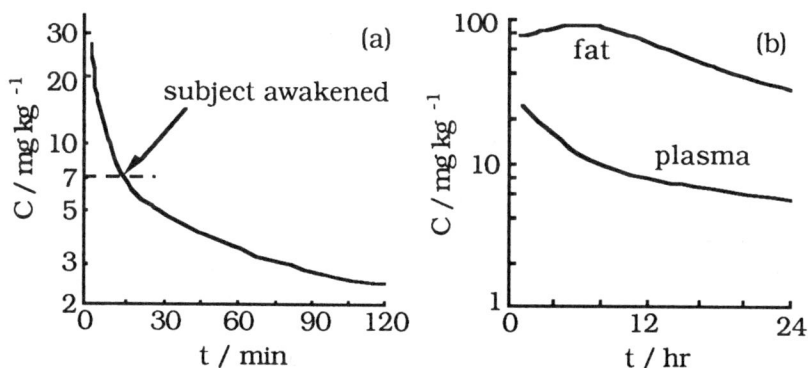

Figure 12.1 Thiopentone plasma concentrations following a single intravenous injection; (a) 400mg into a human volunteer; (b) 25mgkg^{-1} into a dog. Blood concentration is proportional to plasma concentration. Graphs are redrawn: (a) from B.B. Brodie, L.C. Mark, E.M. Papper, P.A. Lief, E. Bernstein and E.A. Rovenstine (1950), *J.Pharmacol.Exp.Ther.*,**98**,85-96; (b) from B.B. Brodie, E. Bernstein & L.C. Mark (1952), *J.Pharmacol.Exp.Ther.*,**105**,421-426.

15 min) which has an apparent half-time of perhaps 4-5 min; and a slower phase taking from 15 min to 4 hr. The second phase is not simply a terminal phase because it is not a single exponential fall towards zero concentration.

The long-time behaviour is better displayed in data obtained with larger doses (see Fig. 12.1b) so that the concentrations in the long tail at the end are big enough to measure. These doses would lead to sleeping times of hours, and presumably for this reason, the data were obtained using dogs. Even 4-5 hours after the dose, the concentration in fat is still rising. Only after 10 hours are the concentrations falling everywhere as in a true terminal phase.

To describe these effects using a physiologically based model, each tissue is assigned to a group according to the time the blood flow would take to remove half the thiopentone within it (see Sections 8.4 and S1.1). Faster removal is favoured by higher blood flow and lower binding per unit weight of tissue. Each group is then represented as a single tissue with an amount of thiopentone and a blood flow that are the sum of those for all the tissues in the group. At least in principle the blood flows can be measured independently of the experiments on thiopentone. The simplified model in Fig. 12.2 using just three groups of tissues is adequate to explain the observations qualitatively.

Thiopentone is usually injected as an initial dose to produce loss of consciousness, followed over a minute or so by the rest of the amount needed to maintain anaesthesia until the administration of the main anaesthetic is stable. **While the thiopentone is being administered** the arterial blood contains a high concentration and (see Fig.12.2a) the concentration in high blood flow tissues including the brain increases rapidly towards that in the blood. **The high concentration achieved in the brain is adequate to produce anaesthesia**. By contrast in low blood flow tissues, the relatively small amount of thiopentone that arrives while the arterial concentrations are high increases the tissue

Figure 12.2 A physiological model for the pharmacokinetics of thiopentone. Blood takes thiopentone to and removes it from the tissues. These are represented in the figure by three groups, lean high blood flow in which concentrations change quickly, lean low blood flow in which the changes are slower, and fat in which the changes are very slow. The heart and brain are part of the group with high blood flow per unit weight, indicated as hbf. Skin and muscle are part of the low blood flow group, lbf. The route of administration is indicated as a syringe injecting fluid into a vein emerging from a tissue in the low blood flow group. Elimination is represented by the pipe emerging from the high blood flow tissues. The diameters of the schematic blood vessels are roughly proportional to the blood flow. The shading in the vessels

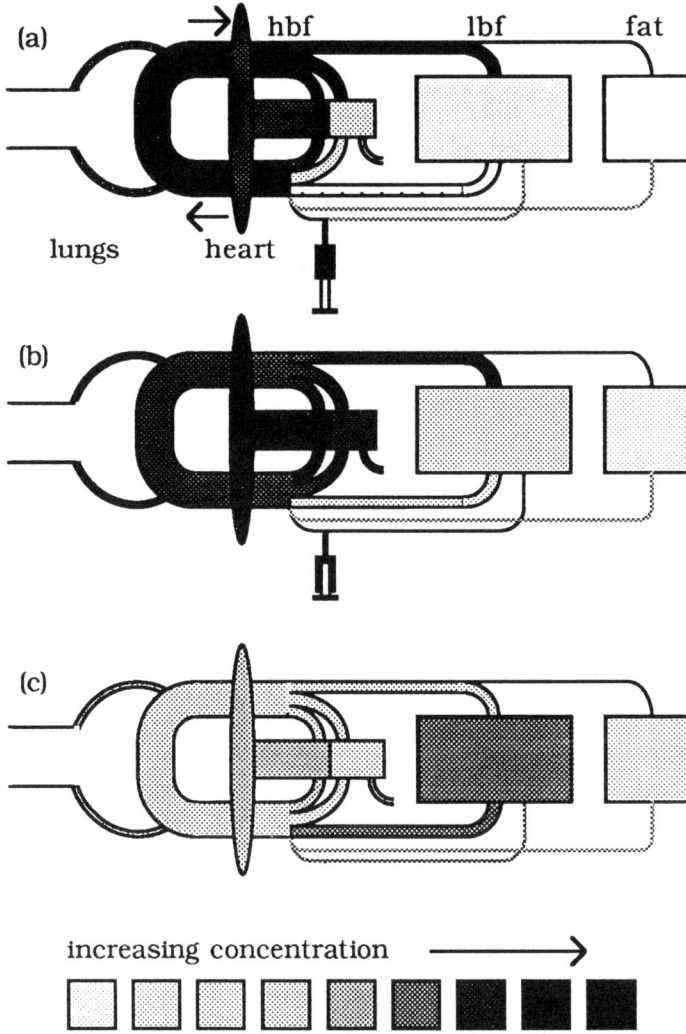

indicates the relative concentration of thiopentone in blood. The shading in the tissues indicates the relative concentration in blood that would be at equilibrium with the tissue. (a) During the injection there is a high concentration in mixed venous and arterial blood which rapidly increases the concentration in high blood flow tissues. (b) In the initial phase after the injection, concentrations in tissues with a high blood flow start falling, those in low blood flow tissues continue rising, and the concentration in arterial blood decreases remaining between the two. (c) In the intermediate phase thiopentone is diffusing out of all lean tissues but into fat. This phase is the last with easily detectable concentrations after a single clinical dose. In the terminal phase (not shown) elimination, primarily in the liver, reduces the concentration in blood and plasma and therefore thiopentone diffuses out of all the tissues into the plasma. As a consequence the concentrations everywhere are falling.

concentration only a little. The different drug concentrations in various tissues mean that the venous blood draining these tissues will have very different concentrations of anaesthetic (see Section S1.1).

Because thiopentone rapidly exchanges between blood cells and plasma, it is convenient in the model to use blood rather than plasma concentrations. Arterial blood is the mixture of the venous blood from all tissues. Thus **during the rapid redistribution the arterial blood concentration, C_b, is intermediate between the concentration in venous blood coming from the low blood flow group, $C_{b,lbf}$, and that for blood coming from the high blood flow group, $C_{b,hbf}$.** If the blood flows are as indicated in Fig. 12.2,

$$C_b = 0.66\, C_{b,hbf} + 0.32\, C_{b,lbf} + 0.02\, C_{b,fat}$$

Over the next 10-15 min (see Fig. 12.2b), **thiopentone diffuses down its concentration gradient out of the brain into the blood while at the same time it is diffusing down its concentration gradient into skin, muscle and fat.** This corresponds to the steepest part of the fall in the plasma concentration vs time curve; it has a half-time of 4-5 min. In practical use if nothing else were done, the patient would wake up after 2-4 redistribution half-times. During this time some thiopentone is being eliminated from the body, by some estimates about 15% is lost, but most of the thiopentone that comes out of the high blood flow tissues is diffusing into other tissues.

At the end of the initial redistribution (see Fig. 12.2c), which corresponds to the knee on the curve in Fig. 12.1a, the concentration in muscle and skin has risen far enough and that in the central organs and blood has fallen far enough for there no longer to be a concentration gradient for movement into skin and muscle. For the concentrations to decrease further the thiopentone must go somewhere else. **The rate of disappearance from the blood is now much less rapid and is accounted for by two routes, transfer into fat and hepatic elimination.** From this time on thiopentone is diffusing out of all lean tissues. After ca 4-8 hr in man, thiopentone is also leaving fat. The relative importance of elimination and redistribution in the time interval between 1/2 hr and about 6 hr is still being debated. Using direct tissue assay in dogs, Brodie's group found over half the dose of thiopentone still in the body after 24 hr, i.e. the terminal half-life in dogs is greater than 24 hr. In Benet & Sheiner's best judgement

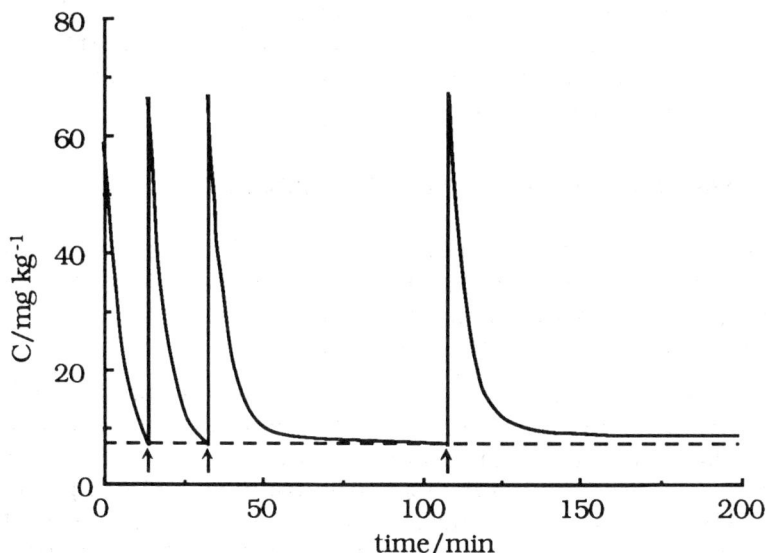

Figure 12.3 The dramatic increase in sleeping time when thiopentone is given repeatedly. The minimum concentration for anaesthesia is indicated by the dashed line. Repeat doses were given at the arrows. (Calculated from Fig. 12.1).

(Goodman & Gilman, Supplement 2), **the terminal half-life for thiopentone in man is *ca* 9 hr.**

Redistribution is crucial in the clinical use of thiopentone. If the initial decrease in concentration following any dose were the result of elimination, then each doubling of the dose would prolong the sleeping time by about a half-life, i.e. a dose 8 times larger would extend sleeping time by 10-15 minutes. However, in fact **at recovery of consciousness after a normal dose most of the thiopentone has not been eliminated, it has only been redistributed within the body. If a substantially larger dose is given, then the concentration after the initial rapid redistribution remains above the level for anaesthesia. Recovery now has to await the much slower processes of redistribution into fat and actual elimination.**

These effects were seen clinically in the 1940s when attempts were made to use thiopentone as the sole anaesthetic. As soon as the anaesthetic effect began to wear off another dose was given, (see Fig. 12.3). With repeated doses, after each dose, the concentration in skin and muscle increases. The redistribution into skin and muscle still occurs, but the rapid fall in concentration now ends at a higher concentration, and following the 4th or 5th dose even after the fast redistribution the concentration is still above the minimum level for anaesthesia. The time to waking is then hours instead of minutes.

12.2 GASEOUS AND VOLATILE ANAESTHETICS

Gaseous and volatile anaesthetics are absorbed into and eliminated from the body via the lungs. Metabolism of these anaesthetics occurs and is important in their toxic effects but it is usually negligible as a route of elimination.

In the steady state the concentrations of the anaesthetic in the air, the blood, and the brain are all at equilibrium with each other. Therefore the steady-state potencies of the anaesthetics could be compared by tabulating concentrations in blood, plasma or the inspired air. The concentration in air is proportional to the partial pressure. By convention **the potency of a gaseous or volatile anaesthetic is defined as the inverse of the partial pressure needed to produce anaesthesia**.

The oil/gas partition coefficient of a substance is defined as the ratio of its concentrations in oil and in the air above the oil at equilibrium, $K_{oil/gas} = C_{oil}/C_{gas}$. As early as 1902 Meyer and Overton observed that the partial pressure needed to produce anaesthesia was inversely proportional to the concentration of the anaesthetic that would dissolve in olive oil at that partial pressure. In other words the potency for volatile and gaseous anaesthetics is proportional to the oil/gas partition coefficient. The implication of this observation is that regardless of the anaesthetic, anaesthesia ensues when the concentration at hydrophobic sites reaches a critical level. These sites appear to the anaesthetic to be like olive oil.

The potency of an anaesthetic does not predict the time course of induction and recovery from anaesthesia. For all the gaseous and volatile anaesthetics in use, concentrations in the brain follow changes in the arterial concentration with only a small lag (see Section S1.1). Thus **induction and recovery are governed by the factors that determine the concentration in arterial blood**.

Elimination of anaesthetic requires that it be delivered to the lungs by the blood, that it cross the alveolar membrane, and then that it is carried out of the lungs in the expired air (see Fig. 12.4). Anaesthetics cross the alveolar/capillary wall rapidly thus the

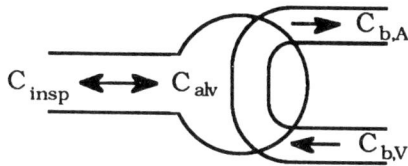

Figure 12.4 Flows and concentrations important in the elimination of gaseous and volatile anaesthetics. The entire cardiac output, c. 5 litre min^{-1} passes through the lungs. Air enters and leaves the lungs at a ventilation rate of about 6 litre min^{-1}. Concentrations in the inspired air and alveolar air are C_{insp} and C_{alv} respectively, those in venous and arterial blood, $C_{b,V}$ and $C_{b,A}$.

concentrations in systemic arterial blood (= pulmonary venous blood) and in alveolar air reach equilibrium,

$$C_{b,A} = K_{blood/gas} C_{alv}$$

where $K_{blood/gas}$ is the blood/gas partition coefficient. In the steady state, there is no net movement of anaesthetic into or out of the body. Thus just as much comes in on each breath as goes out and the inspired and alveolar concentrations are equal. Similarly the concentrations in arterial and venous blood are the same.

At the start of recovery (see Fig. 12.5), the concentration in inspired air drops to zero. The events that follow depend on the blood/gas partition coefficient. When blood arrives in the lungs, it gives up some of its anaesthetic to the alveolar air. **If the blood/gas partition coefficient is small as for ethylene and cyclopropane** (see Table 12.1), then at equilibrium the

Table 12.1 Anaesthetic partial pressures and partition coefficients.

Anaesthetic	pp for anaesthesia /mmHg	$\dfrac{C_{oil}}{C_{gas}}$	$\dfrac{C_{fat}}{C_{blood}}$	$\dfrac{C_{lean\ body}}{C_{blood}}$	$\dfrac{C_{blood}}{C_{gas}}$	
Ethylene	230	1.2	6	1	0.15	
Nitrous oxide	760	1.4	2.3	1	0.47	slower recovery
Cyclopropane	70	11.9	15	1.3	0.55	
Halothane	6	224	65	2	2.4	
Ether	12	65	4.2	1	12	

concentration in the air must be higher than in the blood, so most of the anaesthetic that arrives in the systemic venous blood is released into the air as the concentrations in the air and the blood come to equilibrium. Thus **the air leaving the lungs will contain most of the anaesthetic that arrives in the blood and only a low concentration of anaesthetic will remain in the blood leaving the lungs** (see Fig. 12.5a). Because the concentration of anaesthetic in the blood perfusing the brain is now low, **the concentration in the brain falls rapidly, and recovery occurs within a few minutes**. But note, even though most of the anaesthetic has been washed out of the brain, there is still anaesthetic in muscle, skin, fat, and mixed venous blood (see Fig. S 2.2b). Arterial blood and brain will therefore contain low concentrations of anaesthetic until it is washed out of the rest of the body.

If the blood/gas partition coefficient is large as for ether, recovery follows a different pattern. Now when equilibrium is reached in the alveoli, there is more anaesthetic in the blood than in the gas. As a result **only a small proportion of the anaesthetic that arrives goes out in the air, most carries on into the arterial blood** (see Fig. 12.5c). The arterial concentration is thus only a little below the venous concentration for the anaesthetic. Blood arriving in the brain still has a high concentration of anaesthetic and only a small amount of anaesthetic leaves the brain. **Reduction of the concentration in arterial blood and brain now requires a fall in the concentration in mixed venous blood** (see Fig. 12.5d). The concentration in mixed venous blood falls as the concentrations in all the lean tissues of the body go down. **Thus to reduce the concentrations in arterial blood and brain a major fraction of the anaesthetic present in all lean tissues must be eliminated.** The half-life for this process is determined by the clearance and volume of distribution for the lean tissues.

The lean tissue volume of distribution is almost the same for all the anaesthetics. The half-life varies because the clearances vary. **For large blood/gas coefficients, the rate of excretion is limited by the ability of the expired air to carry the anaesthetic**

Figure 12.5 Simple physiological model for the elimination of an anaesthetic from the body. The tissues of the body are represented as three groups, those with high and low blood flows and fat. The heart and brain are part of the high blood flow group. The diameters of the schematic blood vessels are roughly proportional to the blood flow. The shading in the vessels indicates the concentration of the anaesthetic relative to that in blood at steady state. The shading in the lungs and tissues indicates the relative concentrations in blood that would be at equilibrium with the air or

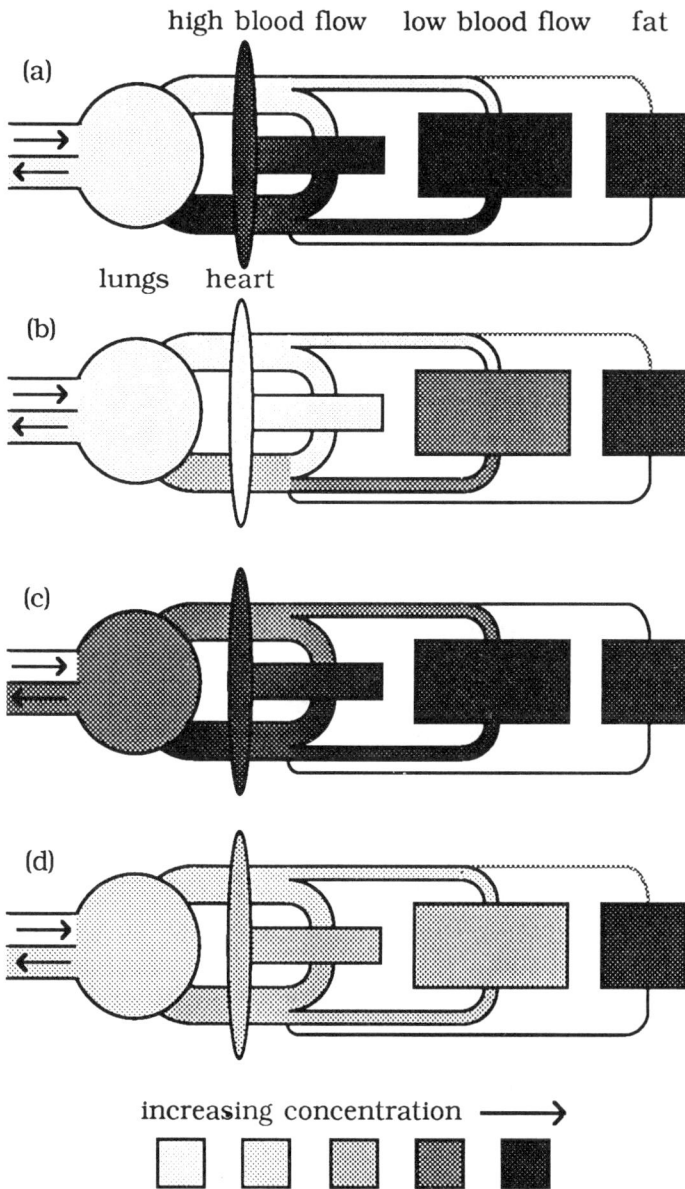

high blood flow   low blood flow   fat

(a)

lungs   heart

(b)

(c)

(d)

increasing concentration ⟶

tissues. (a) & (b) Anaesthetics with small blood/gas partition coefficients; (c) & (d) those with large blood/gas partition coefficients. (a) & (c) indicate the concentrations just after the concentration in the inspired air is reduced to zero. (b) & (d) indicate the concentrations after approximately one half-life for elimination of the anaesthetic from the lean tissues of the body. In (c) & (d) the actual concentrations in air are much less than those in blood.

out of the lungs. For these the larger the blood/gas partition coefficient, the less anaesthetic is expired with each breath and the longer the half-life. For ether with a blood/gas coefficient near 12, the half-life is about an hour. Excretion can be made faster if the ventilation rate is increased by adding carbon dioxide to the inspired air.

If induction were carried out using the partial pressure needed in the steady-state, the time course of the concentrations in the body would be the mirror image of those seen in recovery (compare infusions in Chapter 9). **For $K_{blood/gas}$ small**, little anaesthetic needs to enter the blood to equilibrate it with alveolar air, and thus very rapidly both are near equilibrium with the partial pressure in inspired air, i.e. **induction is rapid. For $K_{blood/gas}$ large**, most of the anaesthetic inspired is transferred to the blood, the partial pressure in alveolar air is thus far below that in the inspired air and the concentration in blood at equilibrium with the alveolar air is thus only a fraction of that needed to produce anaesthesia. **Induction would be slow if the anaesthetist did not use much higher partial pressures in the initial period** (compare Section 9.2).

The concentration of anaesthetics in adipose tissue varies very slowly because fat has a low blood flow per unit weight and it contains a large amount of anaesthetic at equilibrium compared to blood (see Section S1.1). During short procedures the concentrations in fat and in the venous blood returning from it are always low. By contrast after a long procedure the amount of anaesthetic accumulated in fat can be quite large and long after administration is discontinued the anaesthetic concentration in venous blood coming from it is a large fraction of the arterial concentration during the operation. However, the total blood flow through fat is only 2% of cardiac output Thus the anaesthetic removed from the fat produces a concentration in mixed venous blood which is less than 2% of the original arterial level. This low concentration has little effect on the recovery of consciousness, but it does produce a long tail of subanaesthetic concentrations which may contribute to anaesthetic hangover.

PART III
SUPPLEMENTARY TOPICS

The preceding chapters have introduced the fundamentals of pharmacokinetics. Most of the material covered there belongs in any introductory course. The supplements which follow provide more advanced, optional material.

S1 THE TIME COURSE OF DRUG DISTRIBUTION

Concentrations in either plasma or blood are emphasized in pharmacokinetics because these can be measured routinely. However, to reach their sites of action most drugs must be distributed from the plasma to the tissues.

S1.1 AMOUNT AND CONCENTRATIONS IN A TISSUE

For almost all drugs exchange across peripheral capillary walls is rapid. Thus except transiently during rapid changes, the concentration in the venous plasma draining from a tissue and the concentration in the extracellular fluid of the tissue are close to equilibrium with each other. **Furthermore many drugs either don't cross cell membranes or else do so rapidly. For these the amount in a tissue is proportional to the concentration in the venous plasma emerging from it.**

Drug is delivered to the tissues in arterial blood and removed from them in the venous blood. For almost all drugs the rate of removal is proportional to the concentration in venous plasma and to the tissue blood flow. Because the amount in a tissue and the rate of removal from it are both proportional to the venous concentration, they are proportional to each other. The tissue concentration therefore varies in the same manner as the concentration in a beaker (see Sections 8.2 and 9.1). Whenever the arterial concentration is constant, the tissue concentration approaches a steady value exponential:time course of tissue concentrationly with a tissue half-life

$$t_{1/2} = 0.69 \; \frac{\text{amount in tissue}}{\text{rate of removal}} \quad \propto \quad \frac{\text{amount in tissue}}{\text{tissue blood flow}}$$

Because both the amount in the tissue and the tissue blood flow are proportional to the size of the tissue, they are often expressed per kg of tissue. **If the amount in a tissue is large for a given concentration in plasma, then it takes a long time for the blood to deliver or remove enough to change the concentration and the tissue half-life is long. Similarly if the blood flow to a tissue is high, more substance can be removed at any concentration and changes occur quickly, i.e. the tissue half-life is short.**

For any one tissue, the tissue half-life varies from one drug to another because the sites and extent of binding vary. For any one drug, the half-life varies between tissues both because binding differs and because the blood flow per kg varies. For many drugs (usually those with volumes of distribution between 30 and 100 litre, 0.4 to 1.4 litre kg^{-1}), equilibrium concentrations are similar in plasma and the lean tissues. For these, half-lives in tissues with a high blood flow per unit weight of tissue (> 200 ml min^{-1} kg^{-1}) such as heart, viscera, and glands are typically 1-5 min. By contrast resting muscle and cool skin have a much lower blood flow per unit weight (< 50 ml min^{-1} kg^{-1}) and tissue half-lives are typically 20-40 min. Half-lives in brain are short for drugs that can easily cross the blood-brain barrier (see Sections 7.2.3 and 12.1). In adipose tissue the blood flow is very small (< 20 ml min^{-1} kg^{-1}), and for lipid soluble drugs, the equilibrium concentration in the fat can easily be ten times that in blood. For these drugs the half-life in fat can be many hours.

For many drugs and most tissues, when the plasma concentration changes, the tissue concentrations change with only a modest lag. Even for "remote" or "deep" sites at which concentrations may take many dose intervals to rise or fall (see Section S1.2), the average concentration remains proportional to the average plasma concentration.

S1.2   THE CONSEQUENCES OF SLOW TISSUE PENETRATION: GENTAMICIN

Slow penetration to a site of action increases the time required to achieve effective (or toxic) concentrations at the site (see Fig. S1.1). **It can even mean that sufficient concentrations are never reached if there is a mechanism for removing the drug from the region of the site, e.g. by metabolism or by the flow of CSF in the brain.**

Slow penetration and the accompanying slow removal may be suspected first when the drug or a metabolite is found in the urine long after the last dose. It can also sometimes be detected as a long tail in plasma concentration at the end of a series of doses. Such a tail is well documented for **gentamicin**. Following a single dose the plasma concentration falls to low levels and most of the drug is eliminated with a half-life of *ca* 2 hr just as expected for a drug eliminated by glomerular filtration, CL = 90 ml min^{-1}, from a volume of distribution equal to the total extracellular fluid volume, about 16 litres. However, following a series of doses it is apparent that this phase does not continue to completion; it ends with low plasma concentrations that subsequently decline towards zero with a half-life of more than 50 hr. This long, terminal half-life reflects the return of the drug from locations that it could reach only slowly. Following a single dose little gentamicin has reached these deep sites (see

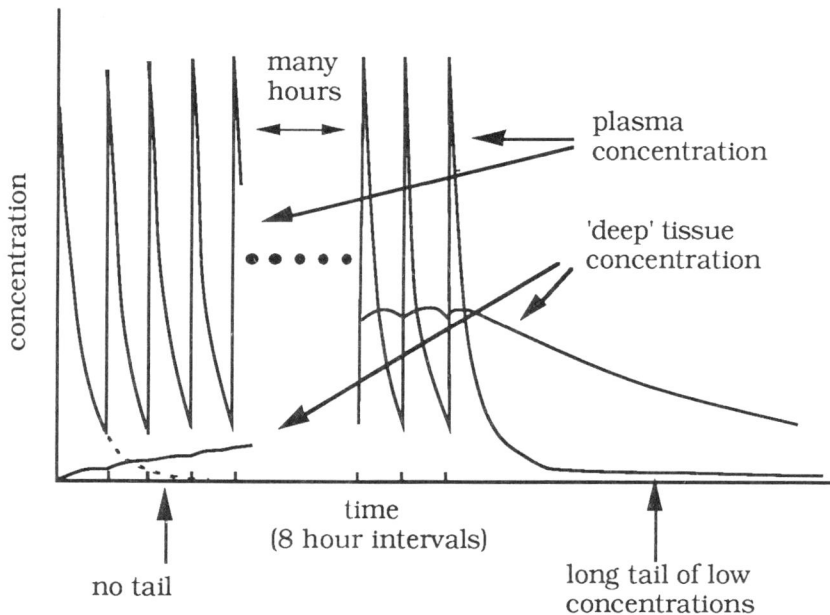

Figure S1.1   Plasma and "deep" tissue concentrations during repetitive dosing. Example loosely based on gentamicin. After a single dose the concentration declines to undetectable levels with a half-life of about 2 hr. After many doses this phase of the decline in concentration ends before the plasma concentration reaches zero. The long tail of plasma concentration, which represents the true terminal phase, occurs because gentamicin is slowly removed from the "deep" tissues by the blood and taken to the kidneys where it is excreted.

Fig.S1.1) and the tail is undetectably small, but after many doses significant accumulation has occurred and the tail is large enough to be measured. For gentamicin accumulation at the deep sites is extensive. This accumulation is important because the toxic effects that limit the use of gentamicin occur at deep sites.

The persistence of low plasma concentrations after most of a dose has been eliminated is sometimes important and sometimes not. In practice, the tail can be ignored in the calculation of pharmacokinetic constants and in their use to design dosage regimens provided: (1) The concentrations are low enough that they don't produce any effects; (2) The area under the tail is negligibly small; and (3) The effects of the drug are not produced at the remote or deep sites. (See Section E.2.10 for a tail which must not be ignored.) When a tail is ignored, the half-life is calculated for the phase of the decrease in concentration that accounts for elimination of most of the dose.   However, the volume of distribution during this phase, calculated as $t_{1/2} \cdot CL / 0.69$, is not actually V_z and it can be substantially smaller than V_{ss}. Just this effect is seen with gentamicin where the volume of distribution during elimination of most of a single dose corresponds roughly to the extracellular fluid volume, which gentamicin reaches and leaves rapidly, while the steady-state volume of distribution is several times larger reflecting the regions that gentamicin can reach only slowly.

The use of data for a test dose of gentamicin to predict the concentrations produced by multiple doses is illustrated in Section E.2.4.

THE CONSEQUENCES OF PLASMA PROTEIN BINDING

Many drugs bind to plasma proteins. Acidic and neutral drugs and some basic drugs, e.g. diazepam, bind primarily to plasma albumin. Most basic drugs bind primarily to an α_1-acid glycoprotein.

Binding to plasma proteins increases the quantity of a drug that can be carried in blood with a free plasma concentration within the therapeutic range. To increase the free concentration in a tissue to an effective level, a quantity of the drug must be carried from the site of absorption to the tissue and it must subsequently be removed to the sites of elimination. If the binding of the drug in the tissue is extensive, the quantity that must be transported can be large compared to the total amount carried in the volume of blood that passes through the tissue in several minutes. For many drugs distribution around the body would be very much slower than observed if binding to plasma proteins did not increase the amount that can be carried. Examples of such drugs include chlorpromazine, desmethylimipramine, diazepam, flurazepam (as its metabolite desalkylflurazepam), haloperidol, imipramine, and propranolol.

Plasma protein binding increases the steady-state total plasma concentrations needed to produce effects. Changes in binding are one, probably a major, source of variation in the relation between measured, total concentrations and therapeutic response and as such they can substantially complicate the use of measured total plasma concentrations for dose adjustment. It is tempting to suggest that if free concentrations could be measured easily they would be more useful than total drug concentrations in plasma as predictors of therapeutic and toxic effects.

Renal failure, cirrhosis of the liver, and nephrotic syndrome can markedly reduce binding to plasma albumin, e.g. for warfarin, diazepam and phenytoin. These changes partly reflect decreased albumin concentration, but in addition in renal failure there also appear to be binding inhibitors.

Renal failure and conditions causing stress such as surgery tend to increase the concentration of the α_1-acid glycoprotein and the binding of basic drugs like propranolol. On the other hand nephrotic syndrome, malnutrition and hepatic disease tend to decrease the concentration and binding.

S2.1   STEADY-STATE CONCENTRATIONS AND CLEARANCE

To produce a change in the steady-state response to a drug, a change in plasma protein binding must lead to a change in the steady-state free concentration of the drug in plasma (but see section S2.3 for a qualification). The change that is produced depends on the mechanism of elimination.

If elimination occurs by glomerular filtration or any mechanism with a low extraction ratio (see Sections 5.2 & 5.3), the rate is proportional to the free rather than the total concentration in plasma. Thus in the steady state because the average rates of absorption and elimination are equal, as long as the rate of absorption is constant, a change in the percentage bound in plasma will have no effect on the average rate of elimination and the average steady-state free concentration. **For any drug eliminated by a mechanism with a low extraction ratio, the dose rate should not be altered in response to a decrease in plasma protein binding even though the conventional clearance will be larger and the total plasma concentration will be smaller. This lower total concentration is just that required to keep the free concentration, $C^{free} = f\,C$, constant.** Drugs with low extraction ratios, extensive plasma protein binding, and critical free concentrations include digitoxin, warfarin, phenytoin, and tolbutamide.

If elimination occurs by a mechanism with an extraction ratio near one (see Section 5.4), the rate of elimination is proportional to the total concentration of drug in plasma or blood, i.e. at least approximately, the clearance is constant regardless of the fraction that is free. Thus the total steady-state concentration produced by a given rate of absorption will remain constant. A decrease in binding at constant total concentration implies an increase in the free concentration and hence presumably a change in effects. It would thus seem reasonable to decrease the dose rate. **Apparently those drugs that have high extraction ratios and extensive binding to plasma proteins either are infused with constant monitoring of effects (e.g. lignocaine) or else don't require sufficiently accurate control of concentration for changes in plasma protein binding to be clinically important.**

S2.2 VOLUME OF DISTRIBUTION AND AMOUNT IN THE BODY.

Even though free concentrations determine the effects of a drug, total concentrations are normally used in pharmacokinetics. The shortcomings of this approach are highlighted by the consequences of changes in plasma protein binding. For any total amount of drug accumulated in the body, if binding to plasma proteins is decreased, the total plasma concentration will be smaller, and thus the volume of distribution,

$$V_{ss} = \frac{\text{total amount in body}}{C}$$

will be larger. However, the total amount that must be accumulated in the body to achieve and maintain a target free concentration is the sum of the amounts in the plasma and the tissues. A reduction in binding to plasma proteins does not itself change binding in the tissues. Thus the total amount to be accumulated in the body to reach a target free plasma concentration is smaller by the same amount as the reduction in the amount bound in plasma. In other words to reach a target free concentration somewhat less drug must be accumulated in the body even though the volume of distribution is greater!

If most of a substance in plasma is free, even large percentage changes in the amount bound in plasma will have little effect on C^{free} or V_{ss}.

If a substance is so strongly bound to the plasma proteins that most of the drug in the body is plasma protein bound, as for warfarin (see Section 7.3.1), then even after the ratio C^{bound}/C^{free} is decreased, most is still bound to plasma proteins and V_{ss} increases only slightly above the volume accessible to the plasma proteins. However, **a reduction in the binding can greatly increase the free concentration corresponding to any total amount in the body.**

By contrast if most of the substance is in the tissues and most of that in plasma is bound, as for benzodiazepines, chlorpromazine, desmethylimipramine, digitoxin, phenytoin and many others, then a decrease in the percentage bound in plasma, b, produces a large increase in the conventional volume of distribution, V_{ss}, but only a small reduction in the amount that must be accumulated in the body to achieve a steady-state free concentration

S2.3   HALF-LIFE

For the same dose and dose interval a decrease in half-life may be clinically significant because it leads to greater variation in concentration between doses.

For drugs that are eliminated by a mechanism with a small extraction ratio (see Section 5.3), **decreased plasma protein binding decreases the half-life but usually not by much.** For a known amount of drug in the body, decreased binding in plasma means that the concentrations in the tissues and the free concentration in plasma are larger. When the extraction ratio is small, this increase in free concentration increases the rate of elimination. Because the half-life is proportional to the ratio (amount in body)/(rate of elimination) (see Section 8.2), this increase in the rate of elimination decreases the half-life. The extent of the decrease varies with the initial distribution of the drug. **When almost all of the total amount in the body is plasma protein bound, a reduction in the amount bound produces** a large increase in the free concentration and **a signficant decrease in the half-life, as seen for warfarin.** (Formally CL is increased with no change in V_{ss}.) **When most of the drug is free or bound in the tissues** then a large percentage reduction in plasma protein binding produces only small percentage increases in the amount bound in the tissues and the free concentration, and **the decrease in half-life is small.** (Formally, CL and V_{ss} are increased in nearly equal proportions.)

For drugs that are eliminated by a mechanism with an extraction ratio near one (see Section 5.4), **decreased plasma protein binding increases the half-life.** A decrease in the bound concentration in plasma decreases the proportion of the drug in the body that is in the plasma, i.e. for a known amount of drug in the body the total plasma concentration is smaller. When the extraction ratio is near 1, this decrease in the total concentration decreases the rate of elimination (see Section 5.3) and hence it increases the half-life. The extent of this increase varies with the initial distribution of the drug. **When most of the drug in the body is in the tissues and most of that in plasma is bound, the effects can be large as seen with propranolol.** (Formally, CL is constant and V_{ss} increases.) Otherwise the effects are small.

S2.4   DRUG INTERACTION BY DISPLACEMENT

Drug interactions can occur by **competition for plasma protein binding**. A significant transient increase in the free concentration is possible if most of the drug in the entire body was originally bound to the plasma proteins. Examples of displaceable drugs with critical plasma concentrations include warfarin and tolbutamide. Any substance, e.g. aspirin or salicylate, that competes for the plasma protein binding sites can displace these drugs. However, fortunately, each of these drugs is eliminated with a low extraction ratio. Thus if the dose rate is unchanged and displacement is the only interaction, in the transition to the steady-state the free concentration will come back to its original value (see Section S2.1). This presumably explains why clinical consequences of displacement are rare.

The important exception is displacment of bilirubin from albumin in the newborn. Bilirubin is the breakdown product of the haem group of cytochromes and haemoglobin. It is present primarily bound to albumin. Elimination depends upon conjugation with glucuronate. This process is usually poorly developed at birth but the rate increases markedly over the next few days. If bilirubin is displaced from albumin before it can be eliminated, the resulting high free plasma concentrations can lead to increased penetration into the brain, deposition in the basal ganglia and permanent neurological damage.

S3: STEADY-STATE VOLUME OF DISTRIBUTION: AUMC

The steady-state volume of distribution is defined as the ratio of the amount in the body, A_{ss}, to the concentration, C_{ss}, during a steady-state infusion,

$$V_{ss} = \frac{A_{ss}}{C_{ss}}$$

But in the steady state the amount in the body also equals

$$A_{ss} = R_0 \, MRT$$

where R_0 is the rate of infusion and MRT, the mean residence time, is the average time that a molecule spends in the body between the moment when it is infused and the moment when it is eliminated (see Fig. S3.1). The rate of infusion in the steady-state is the same as the rate of elimination, i.e.

$$R_0 = CL \cdot C_{ss}$$

Combining these relations, the steady-state volume of distribution is equal to the product of the clearance and the mean residence time

$$V_{ss} = CL \cdot MRT$$

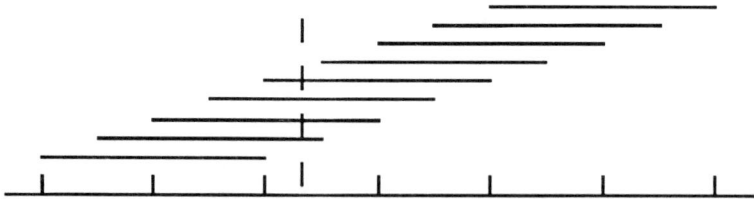

Figure S3.1 A simple illustration of the relation between the rate of arrival, R_0, the mean residence time, MRT, and the number of molecules present at any one time, N. Each line represents a molecule. The line starts at the time when the molecule enters the body and ends when it leaves. At any instant, the number present, i.e. the number which arrived sufficiently recently still to be in the body, is equal to the number of lines crossing that time. This number equals the product of the number of lines to start per unit time, here 2, and their duration, here also 2, i.e. $N = R_0 MRT = 4$. This relation between N, R_0, and MRT is much more general than this illustration. It holds for N and MRT (and to some extent even R_0) equal to mean rather than constant values provided the probability of observing any particular residence time for a molecule is independent of the presence of any others and of the time of its entry.

Both the clearance (CL = DOSE/AUC) and the mean residence time can be evaluated from single dose data. During the infusion or following a single iv injection, molecules of the substance enter the body by the same route and they will eventually leave by the same mechanisms. Thus, provided the fate of any one molecule of drug is independent of the presence of any others, the mean residence time, MRT, will be the same regardless of whether the molecules enter as part of the injection or an infusion. For a single bolus dose with all the molecules entering at t=0, the mean residence time is equal to the mean or average time at which the molecules are eliminated. The mathematical definition for the mean time of elimination, MTE, is

$$\text{MTE} = \frac{\text{Sum}\left[(\text{number leaving in interval } \Delta t \text{ about } t)\, t\right]}{\text{total number that leave}}$$

where the sum includes all intervals for t from zero to infinity. The number that leave the body in the time interval Δt is $CL \cdot C \cdot \Delta t$ (as in Fig. 2.2), while the total number that leave is the number in the dose,

$$D = CL \cdot AUC$$

Thus after a single bolus dose

$$\text{MRT} = \text{MTE} = \frac{\text{Sum}\left[(CL \cdot C \cdot \Delta t) \cdot t\right]}{CL \cdot AUC}$$

On a graph of $C \cdot t$ vs t, the product $C \cdot t \cdot \Delta t$ is the area of a rectangle of height $C \cdot t$ and width Δt. **The entire area under a plot of $C \cdot t$ *vs* t is called the area under the first moment curve or AUMC** (see Fig. S3.3). The sum in the numerator is the clearance times this area, $CL \cdot AUMC$. Thus **for data obtained after a single bolus dose**

$$\textbf{MRT} = \textbf{MTE} = \frac{\textbf{AUMC}}{\textbf{AUC}}$$

and

$$V_{ss} = \frac{D}{AUC}\frac{AUMC}{AUC}$$

AUMC following an intravenous bolus dose (see Fig. S3.2) can be evaluated graphically in the same manner as shown for AUC in Fig. 2.2. The estimate for the area after the last point at time t_1 is $[C(t_1)/\lambda_z^2][1+\lambda_z t_1]$.

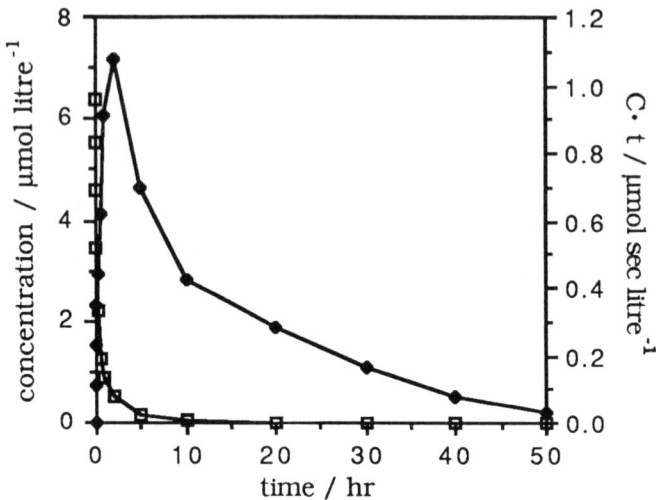

Figure S3.2. Comparison of plots of the concentration versus time (hollow squares) and of the product concentration · time versus time (filled diamonds). The data for methotrexate are taken from Table E.8 . From these it is possible to calculate AUC= 4.07 µmol hr litre^{-1} , AUMC = 15.1 µmol hr^2 litre^{-1}, MPT = 3.7 hr, and V_{ss} = 20 litre. The concentration data can be seen in more detail in Fig. E.2.

V_{ss} can also be calculated from data obtained with a short infusion at a constant rate R_0 lasting from t=0 to t=T. As usual, the clearance is calculated as

$$CL = \frac{D}{AUC}$$

which for a short infusion becomes

$$CL = \frac{R_0 T}{AUC}$$

The calculation of the mean residence time is slightly more complicated because the molecules enter the body over a period of time. The infusion can be regarded as a series of very many equally spaced identical doses, each of size $R_0 \Delta t$. Regardless of which dose they were in, the molecules have a mean residence time in the body equal to MRT. The average time at which molecules from the dose at t_i are eliminated is therefore t_i + MRT. The overall average time at which elimination occurs is then the average value of t_i, which is T/2, plus MRT, i.e.

$$\text{MTE} = \frac{T}{2} + \text{MRT}$$

However, the average time of elimination can still be calculated from its definition as

$$\text{MTE} = \frac{\text{AUMC}}{\text{AUC}}$$

Thus

$$\frac{\text{AUMC}}{\text{AUC}} = \frac{T}{2} + \text{MRT}$$

$$\text{MRT} = \frac{\text{AUMC}}{\text{AUC}} - \frac{T}{2}$$

and **for a short infusion**

$$\mathbf{V_{ss}} = \mathbf{CL} \cdot \mathbf{MRT} = \frac{\mathbf{R_0 T}}{\mathbf{AUC}} \left(\frac{\mathbf{AUMC}}{\mathbf{AUC}} - \frac{\mathbf{T}}{\mathbf{2}} \right)$$

S4 THE DOUBLE EXPONENTIAL APPROXIMATION

It is often possible to adjust the four empirical constants in a sum of two exponentials,

$$C = C_1 e^{-\lambda_1 t} + C_2 e^{-\lambda_2 t}$$

so that a plot of this function looks like or fits the plot of plasma concentration versus time after a single intravenous dose. Estimates of the conventional pharmacokinetic constants can then be calculated from these constants using calculus as follows:

$$t_{1/2,z} = \frac{\ln[2]}{\lambda_z} = \frac{\ln[2]}{\lambda_2}$$

$$\alpha = \frac{D}{AUC} = \frac{D}{\dfrac{C_1}{\lambda_1} + \dfrac{C_2}{\lambda_2}}$$

$$V_{ss} = \frac{D}{AUC} \frac{AUMC}{AUC}$$

$$= D \frac{\dfrac{C_1}{\lambda_1^{2}} + \dfrac{C_2}{\lambda_2^{2}}}{\left(\dfrac{C_1}{\lambda_1} + \dfrac{C_2}{\lambda_2} \right)^{2}}$$

$$V_z = \frac{CL}{\lambda_2}$$

and

$$V_{initial} = \frac{D}{(C_1 + C_2)}.$$

AUMC, called the area under the first moment curve, is the total area under the curve obtained by plotting $C \cdot t$ versus t on linear scales (see Supplement 3). If three or more exponential terms are used to describe the concentrations, the sums, $C_1 + C_2$, $C_1/\lambda_1 + C_2/\lambda_2$,and $C_1/\lambda_1^{2} + C_2/\lambda_2^{2}$ must be extended to include all the terms. λ_z equals the smallest of the λs.

104

S4.1 CURVE STRIPPING AND THE USE OF SEMI-LOG PAPER

The empirical constants in the double exponential are obtained from the experimental data by a process called curve fitting. In practice this is now achieved using computer programs that adjust all of the constants until some measure of the difference between the theoretical curve and the data is mimimized. Curve stripping by hand has been relegated to preliminary calculations and examination questions. Nevertheless it is still useful in that it provides a rough indication of the parameters with a minimum of calculations. The only equipment required is a sheet of semi-log paper or a calculator with logarithms.

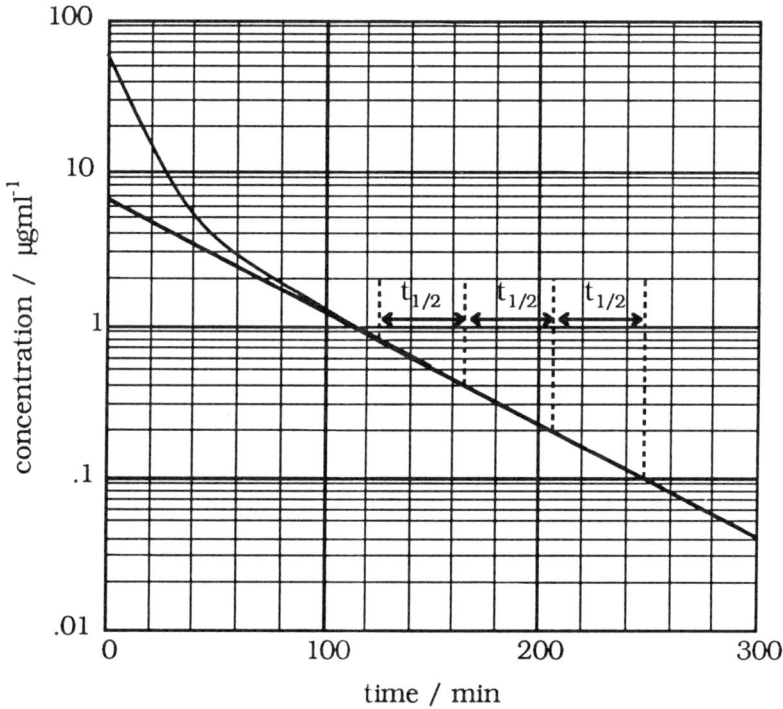

Figure S4.1   The plasma concentrations versus time after an intravenous bolus dose. Time is plotted on a linear scale while the concentration scale is logarithmic. The upper curve is the actual "data" and the lower line is the single-compartment approximation, $C_{sc} = C_z e^{-\lambda_z t}$, where C_z and $\lambda_z = 0.69/t_{1/2,z}$ are calculated as described in the text. The constant value of the half-life in the terminal phase, $t_{1/2,z}$, is indicated by the three arrows. The "data" in this figure are the same as in Fig. 8.1.

Semi-log paper has a logarithimic scale on one axis. Plotted along this scale, concentrations in a geometric sequence, e.g. 1,2,4,8,16,...., will be equally spaced. The logarithmic axis is labelled so that the concentrations divided by some convenient reference value will fit on the scale. For instance in Fig. S4.1 the reference value is $1 \, \mu g \, ml^{-1}$ and at 70 min, $C/1 \, \mu g \, ml^{-1} = 2.22$. The position of the point is interpolated between the scale marks for 2 and 3. At 20 min the value to be plotted is 14.3 and the point is interpolated between 10 and 20.

For data that display a terminal phase the graph on semi-log paper yields a straight line sloping downwards to the right. The equation for this line is

$$\ln[C] = \ln[C_z] - \lambda_z t$$

C_z is easily found on the plot as the intercept on the concentration scale times the reference concentration, i.e. in this example $6.8 \, \mu g \, ml^{-1}$. The terminal phase half-life is determined as the time for the concentration to fall from any starting value along the line to half that value and λ_z is calculated as

$$\lambda_z = 0.69/t_{1/2,z}$$

In Fig. S4.1 the concentration is $0.8 \, \mu g \, ml^{-1}$ at 127 min, one half-life later the concentration is $0.4 \, \mu g \, ml^{-1}$, two half-lives, $0.2 \, \mu g \, ml^{-1}$, and three half-lives $0.1 \, \mu g \, ml^{-1}$. Three half-lives later the time is 247 min. The half-life is thus $(247-127)/3 = 40$ min and λ_z is $0.69/40$ min $= 0.017$ min^{-1}.

Values for $C_1 e^{-\lambda_1 t}$ can be calculated from the data and the terminal phase line as in Fig. S4.2. Draw the curve for the data and a line for C_2 and λ_2 using $C_2 = C_z$ and $\lambda_2 = \lambda_z$. Pick a time t (e.g. 40min), read the value of C from the curve (5.25) and of $C_2 e^{-\lambda_2 t}$ from the line (3.45), subtract one from the other, and plot the difference (1.8). This procedure is then repeated over the entire range of times for which C and $C_2 e^{-\lambda_2 t}$ are clearly different. In the double-exponential approximation the equation for this line is assumed to be

$$\ln[C - C_2 e^{-\lambda_2 t}] = \ln[C_1] - \lambda_1 t$$

The estimates of C_1 and λ_1 are now obtained by drawing a line through the new points. C_1 is the intercept on the concentration scale, times the reference value, in this example $C_1 = 50 \, \mu g \, ml^{-1}$. To calculate λ_1 it is easiest to determine the half-time for the new

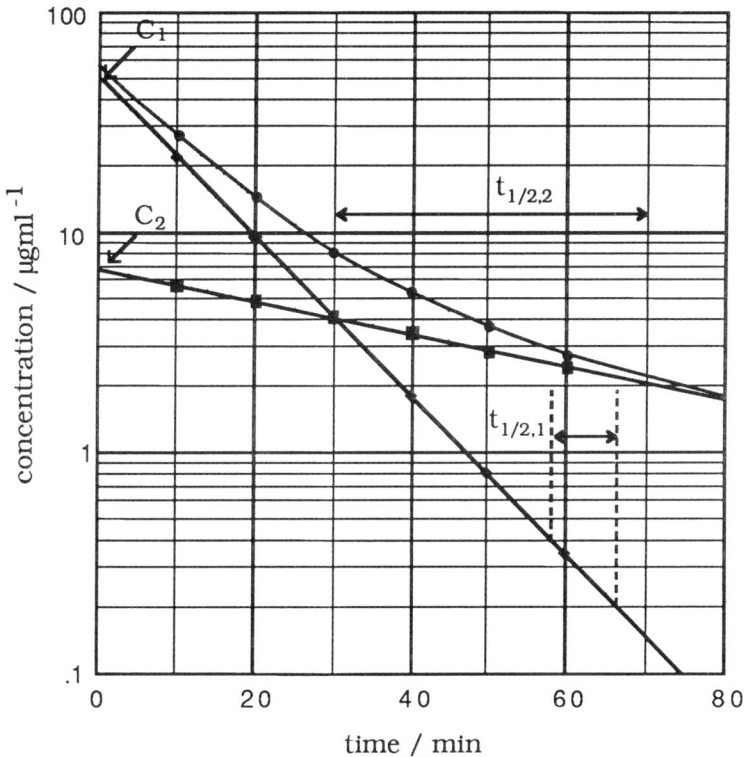

Figure S4.2 The evaluation of C_1 and λ_1 by curve peeling on a semi-log plot. The data represented by the curve and the line drawn for $C_2 = C_2$ and $\lambda_2 = \lambda_2$ are taken from Fig. S4.1. The steeper line and the values for C_1 and λ_1 are calculated as described in the text. The half-lives for the lines are indicated by the arrows. The rate constant for each line is equal to 0.69/half-life.

line, $t_{1/2,1}$ and use $\lambda_1 = 0.69/t_{1/2,1}$. The time for $C\text{-}C_2\mathbf{e}^{-\lambda_2 t}$ to decrease 8 fold from $0.8\,\mu g\,ml^{-1}$ to $0.1\,\mu g\,ml^{-1}$ is 25 min, so $t_{1/2,1}$ is 8.3 min and λ_1 is 0.083 min^{-1}.

If instead of using semi-log paper the data were plotted as ln[C] vs t on linear scales, for each time point it would be necessary to calculate the exponentials of the values of ln[C] and $\ln[C_2\mathbf{e}^{-\lambda_2 t}]$, subtract these values, take the natural logarithm of the answer and plot the final value.

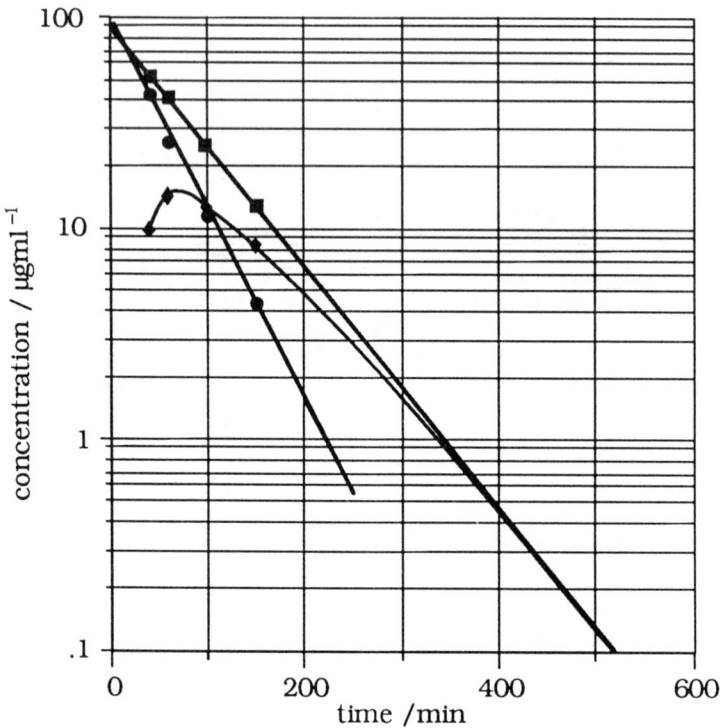

Figure S4.4 Data for 500 mg of dicloxacillin given orally. The analysis of these data to obtain an estimate of the rate constant for absorption is described in the text.

S4.2   THE RATE CONSTANT FOR ABSORPTION

An estimate for the rate constant for absorption, k_{in}, can be obtained from data like that in Table 12.3 using a beaker model. Absorption is assumed to start at a time, t_{lag}, and then to proceed with a rate that declines exponentially with time,

$$R = R_0 e^{-k_{in}(t-t_{lag})}$$

With these assumptions, the concentration in the beaker varies as

$$C = C_0 (e^{-k_{el}(t-t_{lag})} - e^{-k_{in}(t-t_{lag})})$$

where k_{el} is the rate constant for elimination (see Section 8.3).

In Fig. S4.4 the curve connects the data points and the straight line with the smaller slope is drawn tangent to the curve at long times. The half-life calculated from this line as in the preceding section is 53 min. Either k_{el} or k_{in}, whichever is the smaller, can be calculated from this half-life. For these data the terminal phase half-life is almost the same as seen after an intravenous dose (plot the data from Table 12.3), and thus the smaller rate constant is k_{el},

$$k_{el} = \frac{0.69}{t_{1/2 \cdot el}} = \frac{0.69}{53 \, min} = 0.013 \, min^{-1}$$

and the intercept of the line for t=0 is

$$C_0 e^{k_{el}t_{lag}} = 88 \, \mu g \, ml^{-1}$$

The values for C are now read from the actual curve through the data, values of $C_0 e^{-k_{el}(t-t_{lag})}$ are read from the straight line that fits the data for long times, and the values of $C_0 e^{-k_{el}(t-t_{lag})} - C$ are calculated and plotted. For instance for t = 100 min, C = 13 $\mu g \, ml^{-1}$, $C_0 e^{-k_{el}(t-t_{lag})}$ = 24 $\mu g \, ml^{-1}$, and the difference to be plotted is 11 $\mu g \, ml^{-1}$. The best fit straight line is then drawn through the points and the rate constant for absorption is obtained from the slope of the new line,

$$k_{in} = \frac{0.69}{t_{1/2 \cdot abs}} = \frac{0.69}{36 \, min} = 0.019 \, min^{-1}$$

The time at which the two lines intersect, t_{lag} = 20 to 30 min, is the estimate of the time at which absorption starts. These values for k_{in} and t_{lag} needn't be taken too seriously because they are affected by the failure of the beaker approximation during the early part of the data.

S4.3   THE TIME COURSE OF AN INFUSION

A single exponential is much better as a description of the changes at the start and end of a long infusion than as a description of the response to a bolus dose. The underlying reason is that a bolus dose deposits all of the drug in the plasma at one time which produces a large initial peak in concentration. The infusion spreads this one peak into many small ones which makes them less apparent.

The concentrations produced by a constant rate infusion can be calculated using the Principle of Superposition and calculus from the rate of infusion and the concentrations produced by a bolus dose. In effect the infusion is regarded as a series of many small doses whose effects must be added together. If the ratio of the concentration to the dose for a bolus dose is

$$\frac{C}{D} = \frac{C_1}{D} e^{-\lambda_1 t} + \frac{C_2}{D} e^{-\lambda_2 t}$$

the concentration at a time t after the start of an infusion at a constant rate, R_0, is

$$C = R_0 \int_0^t \left(\frac{C_1}{D} e^{-\lambda_1 t} + \frac{C_2}{D} e^{-\lambda_2 t} \right) dt$$

which integrates to

$$C_{ss} - C = R_0 \left[\left(\frac{C_1}{D} \right) \frac{e^{-\lambda_1 t}}{\lambda_1} + \left(\frac{C_2}{D} \right) \frac{e^{-\lambda_2 t}}{\lambda_2} \right]$$

where

$$C_{ss} = \left(\frac{R_0}{D} \right) \left(\frac{C_1}{\lambda_1} + \frac{C_2}{\lambda_2} \right) = \left(\frac{AUC}{D} \right) \cdot R_0 = \frac{R_0}{CL}$$

The fall in concentration at the end of a long infusion is the mirror image of the rise at the beginning. These equations confirm the statement made at the beginning of this section. Because $\lambda_1 > \lambda_2$, the ratio of the constant multiplying the first exponential to that mutliplying the second is smaller in the expression for an infusion than in the expression for a bolus dose.

The concentration a time t after the end of an infusion of duration T is

$$C = R_0 \int_0^T \left(\frac{C_1}{D} e^{-\lambda_1 (t+t_i)} + \frac{C_2}{D} e^{-\lambda_2 (t+t_i)} \right) dt_i$$

$$C = C_1 \frac{1 - e^{-\lambda_1 T}}{\lambda_1 T} e^{-\lambda_1 t} + C_2 \frac{1 - e^{-\lambda_2 T}}{\lambda_2 T} e^{-\lambda_2 t}$$

This time course is intermediate in form between those after a long infusion and after a bolus dose.

S5 COMPARTMENTAL ANALYSIS

It is often convenient to use a series of exponentials to describe or fit experimental data even if only to calculate the conventional pharmacokinetic constants (see Supplement 4). Compartmental analysis attempts to extract more information from the data by using models which explain the need for using two or more exponential terms. These models are based on the assumption that drug molecules in the body can be assigned to one or another of a small number of kinetic compartments. One great attraction of this approach is that it can provide explicit relations for the concentrations in these compartments.

The model-independent approach to pharmacokinetics presented in the rest of this book is relatively modern. From the birth of the subject in the 1930s until the late 1970s almost all attempts to analyze concentration-time curves used compartmental analysis, often in its simplest form, the single-compartment model. Compartmental analysis with two or more compartments is still exploited when, as is usually the case, too little is known to utilize a proper physiologically based model. The relations between the rate constants of compartmental analysis and the conventional pharmacokinetic constants are described in this supplement.

S5.1 THE SINGLE-COMPARTMENT MODEL

The equations of compartmental analysis are written in terms of the amounts of drug present rather than the concentrations. To introduce this approach it is helpful to treat again the single-compartment model that was discussed in Chapter 8.

In the single-compartment model, the body is considered to be a single well-stirred beaker or compartment. In any small interval of time, Δt, the amount eliminated from the compartment is assumed to be proportional to the amount present, A. Thus during intervals when no drug is injected or absorbed,

$$\Delta A = - k_{el} A \, \Delta t$$

where ΔA is the change in the amount within the beaker and k_{el}, the proportionality constant, is called the single-compartment rate constant of elimination. Passing to the limit of infintesimally small intervals

$$\frac{dA}{dt} = -k_{el}A$$

This differential equation can be solved using $dx/x = d\ln[x]$. The solution for any period of time during which no drug is added to the compartment may be written as either

$$A = A_0 e^{-k_{el}t} \quad \text{or} \quad \ln[A] = \ln[A_0] - k_{el}t$$

If a single bolus dose is given at t=0, the initial amount A_0 is equal to the dose.

The amount in the beaker cannot be determined directly by taking small samples of the beaker fluid. The concentration, which can be measured, is related to the amount by the volume of the compartment, V_{sc},

$$C = \frac{A}{V_{sc}}$$

The two constants of the single-compartment model, k_{el} and V_{sc}, are determined from experimental data as described in Chapter 8, i.e. k_{el} is set equal to λ_z.

The half-life is the time taken for the concentration to fall from any initial value,

$$C_i = \frac{A_0}{V_{sc}} e^{-k_{el}t_i}$$

to half that value, i.e. at $t_i + t_{1/2}$ the concentration is $C_i/2$. Thus

$$C_i/2 = \frac{A_0}{V_{sc}} e^{-k_{el}(t + t_{1/2})} = \frac{A_0}{V_{sc}} e^{-k_{el}t_i} e^{-k_{el}t_{1/2}} = C e^{-k_{el}t_{1/2}}$$

that is

$$e^{-k_{el}t_{1/2}} = 1/2 \quad \text{or equivalently} \quad t_{1/2} = \frac{\ln[2]}{k_{el}}$$

As noted in Section 2.6.2, for any beaker model the average concentration during the first half-life is slightly smaller than $3/4\ C_0$. The correct value of the average can be calculated as

$$C_{av} = \frac{1}{t_{1/2}} \int_0^{t_{1/2}} C_i e^{-k_{el}t_{1/2}} dt = \frac{C_i}{k_{el}t_{1/2}} [1 - e^{-k_{el}t_{1/2}}]$$

$$= \frac{C_i}{\ln[2]} [1 - 1/2] = \frac{C_i}{2\ln[2]} = 0.72 \times C_i$$

S5.2   THE TWO-COMPARTMENT MODEL

Supplementary Reference: Riegelman,S., Loo,J.C.K., Rowland,M. (1968), Shortcomings in pharmacokinetic analysis by conceiving the body to exhibit properties of a single compartment, *J.Pharm.Sci.* ,**57**,117-123.

If it is assumed that the initial volume of distribution, $V_{initial}$, corresponds to regions of the body in which the amount present always remains at equilibrium with the concentration in arterial plasma, then these regions taken collectively are called the central or first compartment. The volume of this compartment V_1 is equal to $V_{initial}$ and the amount of drug it contains is $A_1 = V_1C$. The central compartment is always taken to include the plasma and in addition those tissues or parts of tissues in which drug concentrations rapidly come to equilibrium with the plasma. The central compartment normally contains drug located in part or all of the heart, lungs, mesentery, liver, and kidneys, i.e. the tissues with a high blood flow per kg tissue weight. It will also include the brain for drugs that can cross the blood-brain barrier rapidly. For drugs that cross cell membranes slowly, the cell interiors are excluded from the central compartment. Both the intracellular and extracellular regions of skeletal muscles and sub-cutaneous tissues, which have a low blood flow per kg tissue weight, are normally outside the central compartment.

In the two-compartment model all of the drug that has been absorbed but not eliminated is assumed to be in either the central compartment or another peripheral compartment(see Fig. S5.1). It is assumed that drugs are injected into and eliminated from the central compartment and that transfer of drug from one

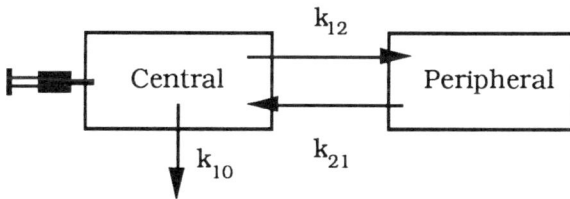

Figure S5.1 The two compartment model. Drugs are injected into and eliminated from the first or central compartment. Transfer of drug from one compartment to the other is assumed to occur at a rate that is proportional to the amount in the compartment of origin and independent of the amount at the destination. The model is completely described by the three rate constants and the volume of the central compartment.

compartment to the other occurs at a rate that is proportional to the amount in the compartment of origin and independent of the amount at the destination, e.g.

$$\text{transfer from 1 to 2} = k_{12} A_1$$

Following a single bolus dose the rates of change of the amounts in the compartments can be written as

$$\frac{dA_1}{dt} = k_{21} A_2 - k_{12} A_1 - k_{10} A_1$$

and

$$\frac{dA_2}{dt} = k_{12} A_1 - k_{21} A_2$$

These equations may be solved by guessing the general form of the solution, plugging this form into the equations above, and, using other information such as the concentrations just after the dose, solving the algebra for the actual values of the constants. The guess work can be avoided by using Laplace transforms. The solution is of the form

$$A_1 = A_{11} e^{-\lambda_1 t} + A_{12} e^{-\lambda_2 t}$$

for the first compartment and

$$A_2 = A_{21} e^{-\lambda_1 t} + A_{22} e^{-\lambda_2 t}$$

for the second. These expressions automatically satisfy the condition that there will be no drug in either compartment a long time after the dose. The additional conditions needed to produce a solution are that initially the entire dose will be in the first compartment,

$$A_{11} + A_{12} = D,$$

and not in the second compartment,

$$A_{21} + A_{22} = 0$$

After inserting the form of the solution into the differential equations, the empirical rate constants, λ_1 and λ_2, can be calculated for any model rate constants as the roots of the quadratic equation

$$(x - \lambda_1)(x - \lambda_2) = x^2 - x(k_{12} + k_{21} + k_{10}) + k_{21} k_{10} = 0$$

The larger root is called λ_1, the smaller λ_2. The coefficients of the exponentials are then

$$A_{11} = \frac{\lambda_1 - k_{21}}{\lambda_1 - \lambda_2} D$$

$$A_{12} = \frac{k_{21} - \lambda_2}{\lambda_1 - \lambda_2} D$$

and

$$A_{22} = \frac{k_{12}}{\lambda_1 - \lambda_2} D$$

In practice of course λ_1, λ_2, $A_{11}/(A_{11}+A_{12})$, and V_1 are determined from the data, for instance by curve stripping (see Supplement 4), and the model constants are calculated from these

$$V_1 = \frac{D}{C(t=0)}$$

$$k_{10} = \frac{\lambda_1 \lambda_2}{\dfrac{A_{11}\lambda_2}{A_{11}+A_{12}} + \dfrac{A_{12}\lambda_1}{A_{11}+A_{12}}}$$

$$k_{21} = \frac{A_{11}\lambda_2}{A_{11}+A_{12}} + \frac{A_{12}\lambda_1}{A_{11}+A_{12}}$$

and

$$k_{12} = \lambda_1 + \lambda_2 - k_{21} - k_{10}$$

The conventional pharmacokinetic constants for a two-compartment system can be calculated from its rate constants and the volume of the central compartment,

$$\lambda_z = \lambda_2 = b/2 - \frac{\sqrt{b^2 - 4k_{21}k_{10}}}{2} \qquad \text{where} \quad b = k_{12} + k_{21} + k_{10}$$

$$V_{initial} = V_1 \qquad\qquad CL = k_{10}V_1$$

$$V_{ss} = V_1 [1 + \frac{k_{12}}{k_{21}}]$$

and

$$V_z = V_1 [1 + \frac{k_{12}}{k_{21} - \lambda_2}]$$

$$= \frac{k_{10}}{\lambda_2} V_1$$

Viewed the other way round it is possible to calculate the constants for the two-compartment model whose behaviour would correspond to any set of the conventional constants,

$$V_1 = V_{initial}$$

$$k_{10} = \frac{CL}{V_{initial}} = \lambda_z \frac{V_z}{V_{initial}}$$

$$k_{21} = \lambda_z \frac{V_z - V_{initial}}{V_z - V_{ss}}$$

and

$$k_{12} = k_{21} \frac{V_{ss} - V_{initial}}{V_{initial}}$$

Because the rate constants and volume in the two compartment model can be calculated from the conventional constants and vice versa, the two sets convey the same amount of information. However, the rate constants carry with them the additional implication that the plasma concentration versus time curve is accurately described by a double exponential. Thus while the conventional constants are couched in terms which remain valid even when the amounts present in various parts of the body vary with different time courses, the rate constants of the two-compartment model are a useful description only when this model actually describes the interaction of the drug and the body. When the plasma concentration is accurately described by a double exponential, most of the drug in the body is in places where the concentration follows the same time course as the amount in one or the other of the compartments. However, because the amount of drug near the sites of action may be a tiny fraction of the total, there is no guarantee that the concentration near these sites will vary in parallel with the amount in either compartment.

S5.3   MULTI-COMPARTMENT MODELS

A double-exponential fails to fit closely the complete concentration versus time curve for most drugs. At least three phases of the kinetics can often be observed, as discussed in detail for thiopentone in Chapter 12. Formally if these three phases are well defined the plasma concentration vs. time after a single intravenous dose can be fitted using three exponentials (see Fig. E.2). However, it is rarely if ever possible to conclude that there are three rather than four or more exponentials in the "correct" description. Compartmental analysis when the plasma concentration vs. time is fitted with n exponentials requires the use of n compartments with at least $2n$ constants. In practice the interpretation of these constants requires a model based on more data than can be obtained from plasma concentration measurements alone. For a simple example of a "physiological" model based on measured blood flows and tissue assays see Chapter 12.

S5.3.1   The Existence of a Terminal Phase and the Principle of Superposition

Provided the rate of each permitted transfer of the drug in the body and the rate of elimination are proportional to the amount present in the region of origin and independent of the amount in the region of the destination, multi-compartment models can mimic the kinetics of a drug to any desired accuracy. Using these models it is possible to prove that there is indeed a final terminal phase in which the amounts and concentrations everywhere in the body are decreasing with the same half-life. Furthermore, in these models, if a dose D_1 produces concentrations $C_{D1}(t)$ and another dose D_2 produces concentrations $C_{D2}(t)$, the concentrations produced if both doses are given are just $C_{D1}(t)+C_{D2}(t)$. This result is a statement of the Principle of Superposition.

GLOSSARY

With a few exceptions, the notation follows the convention most generally accepted in Britain and the United States (M. Rowland and G. Tucker (1980), Symbols in pharmacokinetics, *J. Pharmacokin. Biopharm,* **8**,497-507 repeated as (1982), *Br. J. Clin. Pharmacol.* **14**,7-13). The principal differences are: (1) C^{bound} and C^{free} are used instead of Cb and Cu for the bound and free concentrations in plasma to avoid confusion of Cb with C_b, the total concentration in blood; (2) $C_{av,ss}$ instead of C_{av} stands for the average concentration at steady-state so that C_{av} can be used for the average concentration over any interval; (3) some well known labels are retained from physiology like HBF for hepatic blood flow, RPF for renal plasma flow, GFR for glomerular filtration rate, etc.; and (4) C without a subscript stands for the concentration in arterial plasma because arterial concentrations appear in the theory far more often than venous concentrations. The fact that concentrations are usually measured in venous rather than arterial plasma rarely matters in clinical applications. (At least it is almost always ignored.)

The following is a list of the symbols that are used in equations in Chapters 1-S4. The extra symbols required for compartmental analysis are defined and used solely in Supplement 5. For each symbol a brief description is given followed by the page on which the symbol is introduced or explained.

Subscripts denoting place

A	arterial	lbf	low blood flow tissues
alv	alveolar air	p	plasma
b	blood	rbc	red blood cell
c	central	s&m	skin & muscle
fat	fat	ur	urine
hbf	high blood flow tissues	V	venous
insp	inspired air		

Concentrations without a subscript refer to plasma.

Symbol	Description	Page
A	amount	59
A^-	concentration of the charged form of a weak acid	19
AR	accumulation ratio	78
A_{ss}	amount present at steady-state	100
AUC	area under the curve for a single dose (from t=0 to ∞)	7
AUC_1	area under the curve during first dose interval	77
AUC_{end}	area under the curve after the end of a constant rate infusion	52
AUC_{iv}	area under the curve when the dose is given intravenously	48
AUC_{ss}	area under the curve for one dose interval at steady state (repetitive dosing)	77
$AUC_{t_a}^{\,t_b}$	area under the curve between times t_a and t_b	8
AUC_z	area under the curve, $C_z e^{-\lambda_z t}$	66
AUMC	area under the first moment curve equal to the area under the curve $C\,t$ vs t	101
B	concentration of the neutral form of a weak base	19
b	percentage of drug in plasma that is bound	4
BH^+	concentration of the charged form of a weak base	19
C	total concentration (total plasma concentration in arterial blood unless specified)	4
C_1, C_2	initial concentrations for the exponential components in a double exponential approximation	104
C_{av}	average concentration over an interval of time	8

HBF	hepatic blood flow	34
K	equilibrium dissociation constant	19
$K_{blood/gas}$	gas to blood partition coefficient	90
k_{el}	rate constant of elimination from a beaker model	60
k_{in}	rate constant for absorption	73
$K_{oil/gas}$	gas to oil partition coefficient	90
λ_1, λ_2	rate constants in a double exponential approximation	104
λ_z	terminal phase rate constant	57
M	amount remaining to be absorbed	74
MRT	mean residence time	100
MTE	mean time after the start of dosing at which elimination occurs	101
N	number of molecules	100
pH	$pH = - \log (H^+$ concentration)	19
pK	$- \log$[equilibrium dissociation constant]	19
R_0	constant rate of infusion	9
$R_{av,in}$	average rate of absorption or infusion	7
R_{el}	rate of elimination	11
$R_{el,max}$	maximum rate of elimination	11
R_{in}	rate of absorption or infusion	73
RPF	renal plasma flow	14
T	duration of a short, constant rate infusion	102
t	time	57
τ	dose interval	50
$t_{1/2}$	empirical half life at any time	84
$t_{1/2,beaker}$	half-life of a drug in a beaker model	59
$t_{1/2,in}$	half-life for the rate of absorption	73
$t_{1/2,z}$	half-life in the terminal phase	58

E   EXERCISES AND ANSWERS

Chapters 1-11 emphasize the principles and concepts of pharmacokinetics. This chapter introduces the elementary calculations using clinically important drugs as the examples. After a brief summary of the methods used to calculate the basic constants and a statement of the Principle of Superposition, the rest of the Chapter is organized as exercises and answers. Because calculations are best mastered by doing rather than by reading, the exercises should be attempted before reading the answers.

E.1   CALCULATION OF PHARMACOKINETIC CONSTANTS

E.1.1   Data for single doses

Synthetic, perfect data for practice calculations are given in Tables E.1, E.2 and E.3. Pharmacokinetic constants that can be calculated from them are listed in Table E.4.

Half-life: The terminal phase half-life can be determined from any data that reach a terminal phase by plotting either ln[C] versus time on linear scales or concentration versus time on semi-log paper. The data in Table E.1 for oxacillin are plotted in Figs. 8.1b and S4.1. The methods are described in detail in Chapter 8 and Supplement 4.

Area under the curve: The area under the curve for a plot of plasma concentration versus time is of great importance in pharmacokinetics because it is closely related to both the doses given and the average concentrations that are produced. The area can be evaluated numerically or analytically whichever is more convenient.

   Numerical calculation of the area is described in Fig. 2.2 using the data in Table E.2 for a short infusion of penicillin G. For an intravenous, bolus dose (see Fig. 8.1a) there is an additional practical difficulty. The concentration at t=0 cannot be measured directly and it is difficult to estimate by extrapolation on a linear plot. One approximation is to use a rectangle whose height is the concentration at the midpoint of the first interval. A better procedure is to extrapolate the data to zero time on a log plot (either of Figs. 8.1b and S4.1) and use this value to calculate the area of a trapezoid on the linear plot.

   For many drugs the single-compartment model provides a quick method to obtain an approximate value for the area under the curve by **analytical calculation**,

$$\text{AUC}_{sc} = \frac{C_z}{\lambda_z}$$

For the oxacillin data $\lambda_z = 0.017\,\text{min}^{-1}$ and $C_z = 6.8\,\mu\text{g}\,\text{ml}^{-1}$ (see Fig. 8.1 or Fig. S4.1). Thus $\text{AUC}_{sc} = 400\,\mu\text{g}\,\text{min}\,\text{ml}^{-1}$. In Fig. 8.1a, AUC_{sc} is the area below the lower curve, which is less than half the total. **The single-compartment model is a poor approximation for drugs that are cleared rapidly compared to the rate at which they enter and leave the tissues. Examples of such drugs include the penicillins, lignocaine** (see Section E.2.3) **and methotrexate** (see Section E.2.10). By contrast for drugs that are cleared slowly like digoxin and warfarin, AUC_{sc} is an acceptable estimate of the area (see Sections E.2.2 & E.2.7). The double-exponential approximation for the area,

$$\text{AUC}_{2c} = \frac{C_1}{\lambda_1} + \frac{C_2}{\lambda_2}$$

is discussed in Supplement 4.

Clearance: The clearance is calculated from the total dose, D, given intravenously and the total area under the curve on a linear plot of the resulting concentration versus time (see Chapter 2),

$$\text{CL} = \frac{D}{\text{AUC}}$$

It is important to check that the area is indeed proportional to the size of the dose and thus that the clearance is constant as assumed in this method (see Section 2.3). When the only data available are for doses given other than intravenously, it is possible to calculate CL/F, where F is the availability, but not the clearance.

Table E.1 Simulated plasma concentrations of three penicillins following a 500 mg intravenous bolus dose to human volunteers

Time / min	Concentration / $\mu g\,ml^{-1}$		
	Oxacillin	Penicillin G	Ampicillin
10	27.5	23.0	29.5
20	14.3	11.6	18.3
40	5.3	4.7	9.5
60	2.8	2.8	6.4
80	1.88	1.9	4.8
100	1.26	1.36	3.8
200	0.23	0.25	1.1
300	0.041	0.045	0.34
400	0.008	0.008	0.10

Availability: The availability, F, is calculated by comparing the area under the curve for an intravenous dose with the area under the curve for the dosage form under investigation (see Section 6.3). Practice data are given in Table E.3. (In principle F can be determined after a single dose if the fate of the entire dose can be followed by the analysis of urine, faeces, etc. for both intact drug and all its metabolites.)

Volumes of distribution: The initial volume of distribution, $V_{initial}$, after an intravenous bolus dose is calculated as dose divided by the value of the concentration extrapolated to t=0. An accurate value is rarely if ever needed. The terminal phase volume of distribution, $V_z = V_{area}$, is calculated from the clearance and the half-life (see Section 8.5.2),

$$V_z = \frac{CL \cdot t_{1/2,z}}{0.69}$$

The volume of distribution for intermediate phases is calculated using the same relation, but with the $t_{1/2}$ corresponding to the particular phase (see Section S1.2). When needed, the steady-state volume of distribution can be calculated as described briefly in Table E.4 and in more detail in Supplements 3 and 4.

The rate constant for absorption: When absorption is more rapid than elimination, an estimate for the rate constant for absorption k_{in} can sometimes be obtained by fitting the predicted curve for the concentration in a beaker to the data. The data for an oral dose in Table E.3 is analysed in this manner in Section S4.2. In contrast to the elimination half-life and the clearance, the rate constant for absorption depends on the route of administration and the formulation of the doses.

TABLE E.2 Simulated data for short infusions of penicillin G

Time / min	Concentration / $\mu g\,ml^{-1}$		
	500 mg 40 min	1000 mg 80 min	1000 mg 40 min
10	8.8	8.8	17.5
20	12.9	12.9	25.8
40	16.5	16.5	33.0
60	5.4	18.3	10.8
80	3.0	19.5	5.9
100	1.97	7.4	3.9
120	1.38	4.3	2.8
150	0.83	2.47	1.65
180	0.50	1.47	0.99
210	0.30	0.88	0.60
240	0.18	0.53	0.36
270	0.11	0.32	0.22
300	0.06	0.19	0.13
350	0.03	0.08	0.06
400	0.01	0.04	0.02

TABLE E.3 Simulated plasma concentrations following a single 500 mg intravenous, oral or intramuscular dose of dicloxacillin

Time / min	Plasma concentration / $\mu g\,ml^{-1}$		
	iv	oral	im
0.00			
5.00	82.6		3.1
10.00	61.5		5.2
20.00	37.8		7.7
40.00	20.4	9.5	9.7
60.00	14.2	14.5	10.1
80.00	10.6	14.2	10.0
100.00	8.1	12.7	9.5
150.00	4.2	8.3	7.6
200.00	2.18	5.0	5.7
250.00	1.13	2.8	4.1
300.00	0.59	1.57	2.84
400.00	0.16	0.46	1.31
500.00	0.04	0.13	0.58
600.00	0.01	0.04	0.25
700.00	0.00	0.01	0.11

Table E.4 Pharmacokinetic constants, amplitudes and time constants for the double-exponential approximation. Data for a single, intravenous dose of various penicillins.

	Dicloxacillin	Oxacillin	Ampicillin	Penicillin G
D / mg	500	500	500	500
C_1 / $\mu g\,ml^{-1}$	84	50	40	44.2
C_z / $\mu g\,ml^{-1}$	29.6	6.8	12.4	7.4
λ_1 / min	0.088	0.083	0.077	0.097
λ_z / min	0.013	0.017	0.012	0.017
AUC / $\mu g\,min\,ml^{-1}$	3334	1008	1600	906
AUC_{sc} / $\mu g\,min\,ml^{-1}$	2248	408	1078	449
CL / $ml\,min^{-1}$	156	496	313	552
$V_{initial}$ / litre	4.4	8.8	9.5	9.7
V_z / litre	12	29	27	33
AUMC / $\mu g\,min^2\,ml^{-1}$	183044	31680	100567	31910
V_{ss} / litre	8.9	16	20	19

As described in Supplements 3 and 4, for a bolus dose $V_{ss} = CL \cdot MRT$ where the mean residence time of a molecule in the body is MRT = AUMC/AUC. AUMC is the area under a plot of $C \cdot t$ vs t.

The values in this table are based on the amplitudes and rate constants reported by L.W. Dittert, W.O. Griffen Jr, J.C. LaPiana, F.J. Shainfeld & J.T. Doluisio, (1970) *Antimicrobial Agents and Chemotherapy*, **1969**,42-48. There is considerable variation in the values of the pharmacokinetic constants determined in different studies.

E.1.2   Data for steady-state infusions

When data are available for long infusions the clearance can be calculated from its definition as

$$CL = \frac{R_0}{C_{ss}}$$

The half-life and thus λ_z can be calculated from the terminal phase on a semi-log plot of either C_{ss} - C versus t at the beginning of the infusion or C versus t at the end. The terminal phase volume of distribution then follows as

$$V_z = \frac{CL}{\lambda_z}$$

The steady-state volume of distribution can be calculated from the area under the curve after the end of a long infusion as described in Section 7.1. (AUC_{end} is also the area between the concentration versus time curve and the horizontal line $C = C_{ss}$ at the start of the infusion.)

E.1.3   Data for repetitive dosing

The ratio of the clearance to the availability may be calculated from the dose and the area under the curve for one dose interval (see Section 11.1) as

$$\frac{CL}{F} = \frac{D}{AUC_{ss}}$$

Separate evaluation of the clearance and availability requires data for intravenous doses.

Provided the dose interval is long enough for the fall in concentration to reach the terminal phase, the half-life can be evaluated from the slope of this portion of a log plot of the concentration versus time, i.e. if t_1 and t_2 are times during the terminal phase

$$C_2(t_2) = C_1(t_1)e^{-\lambda_z(t_2 - t_1)}$$

$$\lambda_z = \frac{1}{t_2 - t_1} \ln \frac{C_1(t_1)}{C_2(t_2)}$$

and

$$t_{1/2,z} = \frac{0.69}{\lambda_z}$$

The terminal phase volume of distribution is calculated as

$$V_z = \frac{CL}{\lambda_z}$$

The steady-state volume of distribution can be calculated from a previously determined value of the clearance and the total area under the curve starting just after the last dose of a long series (compare Section 7.1).

E.1.4   Percentage bound in plasma

Drugs in solution in plasma are either in free solution or bound to the plasma proteins. These forms can be separated by ultrafiltration without disturbing the binding equilibrium. Alternatively the binding can be characterized by equilibrium dialysis with plasma inside the dialysis tubing and known drug concentrations in the (possibly artificial) ultrafiltrate of plasma on the outside. The conventional pharmacokinetic constants are all based on total concentrations.

E.2   CALCULATION OF DOSES, CONCENTRATIONS AND CONSTANTS

Perhaps the most common of all clinical pharmacokinetic calculations is the scaling of doses using **ratio and proportion**. This is an example of the **Principle of Superposition** for drugs that obey linear kinetics. For these drugs the concentrations are proportional to the size of the doses. If a dose D_1 gives concentrations $C_1(t)$, then a dose D_2 differing only in size will yield concentrations

$$C_2(t) = \frac{D_2}{D_1} C_1(t)$$

Furthermore if two doses, D_1 and D_2, are given at different times the concentration is just the sum of those that would be produced if each dose were given alone,

$$C(t) = C_1(t) + C_2(t).$$

Similarly the average concentrations produced by two different dose rates are related by

$$C_{2,av} = \frac{DR_2}{DR_1} C_{1,av}.$$

Help with the exercises can be found in the sections indicated in parentheses. Answers are given in Section E.3.

E.2.1   Lithium: Dose adjustment in response to measured concentrations

Lithium is an example of a drug whose dosage is determined and adjusted based on monitored plasma concentrations. It is used to relieve the symptoms of manic-depression. The dosage must be carefully controlled to minimize side effects and avoid toxicity. Nausea, vomiting, abdominal pain, and renal impairment can occur with peak concentrations as low as $1.5\,mmol\,litre^{-1}$ and severe intoxication involving muscular rigidity, apathy, stupor and coma can occur at concentrations exceeding $3\,mmol\,litre^{-1}$. In some patients lithium induces nephrogenic diabetes at even lower concentrations.

Typical values of the clearance and half-life are $0.35\,ml\,min^{-1}\,kg^{-1}$ and $22\,hr$ respectively. Lithium is almost completely absorbed from oral doses.

The therapeutic effect is presumably related to the average plasma concentration and thus in principle dose adjustment should be based on determinations of the clearance. A test dose of $20.3\,mmol$ lithium has been given to a patient and the plasma conçentration measured at the times indicated in Table E.5. The patient drank a litre of water half and hour before the dose to increase urine flow rate and voided completely just before the dose was given. The urine was subsequently collected just after each plasma sample and the average rate of lithium excretion calculated as amount of lithium collected divided by the time elapsed since the preceding sample.

1) Calculate the half-life, total clearance and renal clearance. (Sections 2.3 and 3.1). What dose rate would yield an average plasma concentration of $1\,mmol\,litre^{-1}$? (Section 11.1).

2) To minimize the cost and the inconvenience to the patient plasma concentration monitoring is based on a single sample taken at a defined stage of the dose cycle.

Table E.5 Plasma concentration and average rate of renal excretion after an oral dose of 20.3 mmol lithium.

time / hr	plasma concentration / mmol litre^{-1}	average rate of excretion / mmol hr^{-1}
0.5	0.44	0.25
1	0.67	0.57
2	0.81	0.77
5	0.61	0.73
10	0.38	0.48
20	0.26	0.31
30	0.21	0.23
40	0.17	0.19
60	0.10	0.13
80	0.067	0.084
100	0.042	0.053
120	0.027	0.034

Values based on data reported by U. Groth, W. Prellwitz & E. Jähnchen, (1974), Estimation of pharmacokinetic parameters of lithium from saliva and urine, *Clin. Pharmacol. Ther.*, **16**, 490-498.

Conventionally for lithium this is just before the next dose on a standard 12 hr cycle. Why is the sample taken at this time? In qualitative terms how will this sample concentration be related to the average?

3) Successful treatment normally requires minimum concentrations in the range from $0.6\,mmol\,litre^{-1}$ to $1.2\,mmol\,litre^{-1}$. Calculate the dose to obtain a target minimum concentration of $0.6\,mmol\,litre^{-1}$, if the measured steady-state (12 hr) concentration after 20.3 mg doses is $1.5\,mmol\,litre^{-1}$.

E.2.2   Digoxin: maintenance dose, loading dose, dose interval, superposition, use of creatinine clearance

Digoxin can be used to produce a positive inotropic effect in the treatment of congestive heart failure or to reduce ventricular rate when this has been disturbed by atrial flutter. The minimum plasma concentrations for these effects are about $0.8\,ng\,ml^{-1}$ and $1.3\,ng\,ml^{-1}$ respectively, but there are large variations between patients. Toxic effects occur even at these concentrations and 50% of patients have drug induced dysrhythmias by $2.5\,ng\,ml^{-1}$. With reduced renal function the clearance and the volume of distribution for digoxin both decrease while the half-life is increased. However, even after allowing for these effects, ca 30% variations are common.

Properties of digoxin (for "average patients"):
With creatinine clearance CL_{Cr} expressed in $ml\,min^{-1}\,kg^{-1}$
    Clearance: $CL = (0.88\,CL_{Cr} + 0.33)\,ml\,min^{-1}\,kg^{-1}$ Half-life: $t_{1/2} = 110\,hr/(1 + 1.2\,CL_{Cr})$
Tablet sizes: $62.5\,\mu g$, $125\,\mu g$ and $250\,\mu g$ Availability: 0.7
Time to peak effect: 30-60 min after i.v. dose; c. 1.5 hr after an oral dose
Only a small proportion of the elimination occurs before the terminal phase.

(1) Calculate an acceptable (practical) dose and dose interval to maintain plasma concentration within the range $1\,ng\,ml^{-1}$ to $1.8\,ng\,ml^{-1}$ for an "average" patient with normal renal function and body weight ($CL_{Cr} = 1.45\,ml\,min^{-1}\,kg^{-1}$, 70 kg). (Sections 11.1 and 11.3).

(2) If $375\,\mu g$ digoxin were given once daily to the same patient, predict the number of doses required for the concentration to first exceed $1\,ng\,ml^{-1}$ and the number of doses given before it last falls below this value. (Fig. 11.3). What are the implications of the calculations in (1) and (2) for the timing of clinical assessment of the treatment?

(3) For the same patient predict a loading dose that would produce digoxin concentrations within the therapeutic range throughout the first dose interval. (Sections 11.2 and 11.5, Fig. 11.3). How can the uncertainties caused by individual variations be taken into account in the loading procedure?

(4) A manufacturer's data sheet recommends that rapid "digitalization" (usually for reduction of ventricular rate) should be carried out with an initial dose of $10\,\mu g\,kg^{-1}$ to $20\,\mu g\,kg^{-1}$ followed by $3.5\,\mu g\,kg^{-1}$ given 6-hourly until the optimal response is reached. Thus the initial doses are scaled in proportion to body weight. Using this procedure a patient with normal renal function has been digitalized with a total loading dose of $1250\,\mu g$. The size of this loading dose conveys information about the interaction of digoxin with $this$ patient. How can this information be used to predict the maintenance dose? How would the prediction differ if the creatinine clearance were $0.5\,ml\,min^{-1}\,kg^{-1}$? (Sections 11.2 and 11.5, Fig. 11.3).

E.2.3   Lignocaine: loading procedure, failure of the beaker approximation

The calculation of loading doses for lignocaine provides an important exception to the rule that the details of the change in plasma concentration after a dose are not important. In this exercise the defect inherent in the beaker approximation is illustrated by calculating the concentrations produced by the combination of a loading dose and a constant rate infusion.

Using a beaker model with $t_{1/2} = 110\,min$ and $CL = 650\,ml\,min^{-1}$, calculate the maintenance infusion rate and the initial loading dose to achieve and maintain a plasma concentration of $2.65\,\mu g\,ml^{-1}$. (Chapter 9). Also calculate or plot the variation in concentration when the loading dose and infusion are given together. Compare the resulting curve with Fig. 9.2. **Why would it be dangerous to administer a loading dose of this size to a patient?**

E.2.4   Gentamicin: plasma concentration monitoring

Dosage regimens for the aminoglycoside antibiotics are designed to achieve sufficient peak concentrations to be bactericidal while keeping the average concentration as low as possible to minimize toxicity. Dosage is adjusted so that the peak concentration (measured 1 hr after a short infusion or intramuscular injection) is within a target range and the minimum or trough concentration is below a ceiling. For gentamicin the range is $5\,\mu g\,ml^{-1}$ to $10\,\mu g\,ml^{-1}$ and the ceiling is $2\,\mu g\,ml^{-1}$.

An intramuscular injection of $1.5\,mg\,kg^{-1}$ has produced measured concentrations of $12\,\mu g\,ml^{-1}$ at 1 hr and $5\,\mu g\,ml^{-1}$ at 8 hr. Suggest a modified dose and dose interval. Assume that the concentration falls exponentially with time from 1 hr after a dose until the next dose. N.B. no assumption is required about the form of the variation during the hour between the dose and the peak sample. (Section 11.3 and ratio and proportion).

E.2.5   Phenytoin: non-linear elimination; fine dose adjustment, drug interactions

Phenytoin is an anticonvulsant used in long term prophylactic treatment of partial and generalized tonic-clonic epileptic seizures. Unfortunately it has toxic effects at concentrations only marginally higher than required to prevent seizures. Furthermore it is eliminated by metabolism that saturates in the same range of concentrations. This combination of properties is dangerous and it is now routine to monitor phenytoin plasma concentration as an aid to the initiation and maintenance of correct dosage. The following exercises illustrate some of the properties of a drug with saturable elimination.

A 50 kg patient is receiving $300\,mg\,day^{-1}$ phenytoin divided into three doses. Assume for this patient that

$$\text{rate of elimination} = \frac{7.5\,mg\,kg^{-1}\,day^{-1} \cdot C}{C + 5.7\,\mu g\,ml^{-1}}.$$

Phenytoin is available in 25 mg, 50 mg and 100 mg tablets.

(1) Assuming that the volume of distribution is constant at $0.64\,litre\,kg^{-1}$, estimate the average, maximum and minimum concentrations produced at steady-state. (Hints: What must be true at steady-state even for non-linear elimination? What is the increase in concentration following a dose?)

(2) What dose rate would produce an average concentration twice as large? **Why is a tablet available that contains a dose that is so small compared to the amount given daily?**

(3) If the dose rate is increased by 25% to $375\,mg\,day^{-1}$ by what percentage per day does the concentration increase for the first few days? How far will it eventually increase? **What are the implications of these observations for patient monitoring?**

(4) When a single agent fails to eliminate convulsions, combinations of two are sometimes tried. Carbamazepine and phenobarbitone are inducers of hepatic metabolism of drugs, including phenytoin. How does this induction complicate the use of either of these agents in combination with phenytoin?

(5) A number of agents including metronidazole, chloramphenicol and cimetidine can inhibit hepatic metabolism of phenytoin. Starting from the conditions stated above what change in plasma concentration would result if the maximum rate of elimination were reduced from $7.5\,mg\,kg^{-1}\,day^{-1}$ to $7.0\,mg\,kg^{-1}\,day^{-1}$? What reduction in dose rate would be required to restore the concentrations to the previous value?

E.2.6   Dicloxacillin

Suggest an explanation for the difference between the pharmacokinetic constants for dicloxacillin and the other three penicillins in Table E.4. (Sections 3.2, 7.3 and S2).

E.2.7 Warfarin: delayed response, loading procedure

Supplementary References:

Fennerty,A., Dolben,J., Thomas,P., Backhouse,G., Bentley,D.P., Campbell,I.A. & Routledge,P.A. (1984), Flexible induction dose regimen for warfarin and prediction of maintenance dose, *Br.Med.J.* ,**288**,1268-1270.

Nagashima,R., O'Reilly,R.A. & Levy,G. (1969), Kinetics of pharmacologic effects in man: The anticoagulant action of warfarin, *Clin.Pharmacol.Ther.* ,**10**,22-35.

Sawyer,W.T.(1983), Warfarin. In: *Applied Clinical Pharmacokinetics*, Ed. D. Mungall, Raven Press, New York, pp. 187-222.

Shetty,H.G.M., Fennerty,A.G. & Routledge,P.A. (1989), Clinical pharmacokinetic considerations in the control of oral anticoagulant therapy, *Clin.Pharmacokin.* , **16**,238-253.

Warfarin is an oral anticoagulant used primarily to reduce the probability of clot formation within the blood vessels. It inhibits reduction of vitamin K epoxide which is necessary for the reuse of the vitamin K in the synthesis of blood coagulation factors II, VII, IX, and X. With normal levels of vitamin K the rate of synthesis of these factors rapidly comes to a new level whenever the warfarin concentration changes. However, even total block of synthesis cannot produce an immediate change in the ability of the blood to clot because the concentrations of the factors can only fall as fast as they are degraded. The half-lives for the fall in concentration range from 6 hr for factor VII to more than 60 hr for factor II. The intended antithrombotic effect develops with an apparent half-life of about 20 hr.

Warfarin dosage must be adjusted accurately. Because the consequences of errors can be severe, the final adjustments must be made at steady-state and in many instances the patients remain hospitalized until stable effects are obtained. Thus there is a premium on procedures which allow the steady state to be achieved as rapidly as possible.

Even at steady state, the relation between warfarin concentration and the antithrombotic effect is variable, depending on factors such as the vitamin K content of the diet, rate of metabolism of the coagulation factors in the liver, and the extent to which warfarin is bound to plasma proteins. Thus **plasma concentration can not be relied upon to provide a reliable guide to dosing.** Fortunately procedures have been developed which allow adjustment using *in vitro* assays. These assays are based on determining the time required for clot formation in a mixture of a blood sample and a reagent containing everything needed for clotting except the factors to be assayed. The results can be reported as the time required for clots to form, as the ratio of the clotting time to that for control samples, or as the dilution of control plasma that produces the same clotting time as the sample. The ratio method of reporting has now been standardized as the International Normalized Ratio or INR. The assays are imperfect in that they assess extravascular coagulation rather than tendency for formation of intravascular clots but, at least in the steady-state, there is a good correlation between these effects.

While measured plasma concentrations are not used to adjust dosage for warfarin, a knowledge of how they vary is essential if the rationale behind the adjustment procedures is to be understood. The following exercises outline a simplified version of an already simplified account. They are intended solely to illustrate the principles and not as instruction in the use of warfarin. For the purposes of this example the four clotting factors are replaced by a single "clotting factor activity" or Act.

In a particular typical patient:

Clotting factor activity, Act, is to be reduced to 20% of the control value, corresponding to an INR of 2.0. The steady-state concentration at which this reduction occurs is $1.2\,\mu g\,ml^{-1}$. It is assumed that warfarin does not affect the processes which degrade the clotting factor activity. Thus this level of activity also corresponds to 80% inhibition of the rate at which the factor activity is synthesized.

After total block of synthesis the clotting factor activity decays with a half-life of 20 hr.

The clearance for warfarin is $180\,ml\,hr^{-1}$ and the half-life 37 hr. Absorption is much more rapid. In the UK the doses available increase in increments of 1 mg.

Variability between patients affects the synthetic activity present, the half-life for decay of clotting factors, the percentage of the warfarin in plasma that is bound, and the clearance of warfarin (the volume of distribution is relatively constant).

A beaker model may be used.

(1) For this patient, what dose rate is required at steady-state? Suggest a dose and dose interval. (Sections 11.1 and 11.3).

(2) If dosing were started at this dose rate when would the concentration first reach $1 \, \mu g \, ml^{-1}$? Approximately when would the average concentration reach the same value? (Figs 11.1 & 11.3). The changes in the concentrations of the clotting factors and hence the antithrombotic effect lag behind these concentrations by many hours.

(3) As the objective is to achieve a given level of clotting factor activity rather than of warfarin, one strategy used in the past was to deplete the clotting factors as rapidly as possible by totally inhibiting synthesis with a large loading dose of warfarin. If an initial dose of 75 mg were given, for how long would the synthesis of clotting factor activity remain below 20% of control? (Section 8.3). If, as a result of variability between patients, synthesis were to remain negligible for this entire period, how much clotting factor activity would remain? This procedure has been abandoned because there is too much risk of haemorrhage.

(4) & (5) These items investigate the extent to which different degrees of inhibition of synthesis affect the initial stage of the decrease in clotting factor activity and the final approach to the target value. Assume that the rate of degradation of activity is proportional to the activity remaining. (Sections 8.3 and 9.1.2).

(4) Compare the reduction in clotting factor activity 24 hr after the start of treatment (initial value 100%) if the rate of synthesis is reduced from 100% to 0% with the reduction if the rate is reduced from 100% to 10% of the initial value.

(5) Compare (a) the time taken for clotting factor activity to reach 25% from a starting value of 40% if the rate of synthesis is constant at 10% of control with (b) the time taken if the rate is constant at 20% of control. What are the implications of these calculations?

(6) In current practice a loading dose roughly twice the anticipated maintenance dose is used for two or three days followed by dose reduction based on the prothrombin time. Calculate the expected maximum and minimum concentrations after each dose for the sequence, three 10 mg doses followed by three 5 mg doses. (Figs. 11.1 and 11.3).

(7) **What are the implications of the variability between patients for the choice of loading doses and the design of a procedure for dose adjustment?:**

E.2.8   Tricyclic antidepressants: correlation of effects with plasma concentration? A cautionary tale

Supplementary References:

Guthrie,S., Lane,E.A. & Linnoila,M. (1987), Monitoring of plasma drug concentrations in clinical psychopharmacology, In *Psychopharmacology: The Third Generation of Progress*, Ed. H.Y. Meltzer, Raven Press, New York, pp.1323-1338.

Amsterdam,J., Brunswick,D. & Mendels,J. (1980), The clinical application of tricyclic antidepressant pharmacokinetics and plasma levels, *Am.J.Psychiatry*, **137**,653-662.

Rudorfer,M.V. & Potter,W.Z. (1987), Pharmacokinetics of antidepressants, In *Psychopharmacology: The Third Generation of Progress*, Ed. H.Y. Meltzer, Raven Press, New York, pp.1353-1363.

The tricyclic antidepressants produce a marked inhibition of noradrenaline uptake into nerve terminals which increases noradrenaline levels in the surrounding region. However, while the uptake block is immediate, the relief of depression develops over weeks of continued treatment. To explain this discrepancy it has been proposed that secondary long-term consequences of the elevated levels are responsible for the antidepressant effects. The fraction of patients deemed suitable for treatment who benefit, and for whom the treatment is therefore continued, varies from 35% to 70% in different studies.

The tricyclic antidepressants are extensively plasma protein bound. They have clearances up to $1100 \, ml \, min^{-1}$, very large volumes of distribution and half-lives longer than 16 hr. First-pass elimination can reduce the oral availability to less than half. Demethylation of the tertiary amine compounds, imipramine and amitriptyline, produces active metabolites, desmethylimipramine and nortriptyline respectively. Both the tertiary and secondary amines can be hydroxylated to products which are known to block noradrenaline uptake. Conjugation of these metabolites with glucuronide renders them inactive.

Because the response to a dose rate varies greatly between patients, it is common practice gradually to increase the dosage of tricyclic antidepressants until a satisfactory result is obtained or side effects intervene. This process is slow and a reliable guide for more rapid adjustment would be welcome. As techniques to measure plasma concentrations of antidepressants have been developed, it has become clear that as a result of differences in the rate of metabolism the same dose can produce steady-state plasma concentrations that vary by as much as fivefold between patients. This large range invites the hypothesis that differences in concentration account for the variability in response. If so the response should correlate much more closely with plasma concentration than with the daily dose. This prediction has been assessed in clinical trials in which a fixed dose rate was used for many patients. For imipramine and nortriptyline definite correlations between effect and· plasma concentration have been found, but for amitriptyline several influential studies have. found no correlation of clinical effect with either the concentration of amitriptyline or the sum of the concentrations of amitriptyline and nortriptyline.

Suggest possible causes for a lack of correlation between plasma concentration (at constant dose rate) and therapeutic response. (For hints: see Sections 1.1.3, 4.6, 5.2, 5.4 and 7.2.3, and Supplement 2). What further investigations might identify which of these causes are important? What role should plasma concentration measurements have in current use of the tricyclic antidepressants?

E.2.9   Theophylline: controlled release, superposition, AUC, half-life

Theophylline is used to produce bronchodilation in the treatment óf severe asthma. Unfortunately it has many side effects. Like caffeine, it can produce marked CNS and cardiac stimulation at concentrations even below the clinical range. Nausea and vomiting can occur at concentrations as low as $15 \mu g\,ml^{-1}$ and at higher concentrations it can produce convulsions and cardiac dysrhythmias.

Both the plasma concentrations and the effects produced by standard doses differ markedly between patients. Fortunately the plasma concentration correlates well with the effects, and plasma concentration monitoring can be used in dose adjustment. The therapeutic range is normally taken to be between $10 \mu g\,ml^{-1}$ and $20 \mu g\,ml^{-1}$ with trough concentrations below $13 \mu g\,ml^{-1}$. Theophylline is rapidly absorbed from conventional oral doses with an availability greater than 90%.

Because the acceptable range of concentrations is narrow and the half-life can be short, a number of controlled or sustained release preparations are available. Experimental plasma concentrations measured after a conventional 400 mg dose of theophylline or a 400 mg controlled release preparation are listed in Table E.6 and plotted in Fig. E.1 together with a simulation for an "ideal" 12 hr controlled release tablet. Normal tablet sizes are 125 mg for conventional doses and 300 mg or 400 mg for the sustained release preparation. The "ideal" tablet releases 400 mg at a constant rate over 12 hr. Assume that the kinetics are linear.

(1) Calculate the terminal phase rate constant and the ratio of the clearance to the availability for the conventional dose and the controlled release preparation? (Sections E.1, 8.1 and 8.2). What would the average concentration be if 400 mg were given once each 12 hr or 800 mg once each 24 hr? (Section 11.1). How would this average differ if the clearance were twice or half the calculated value?

(2) Calculate the plasma concentrations expected if each of these types of dose were given repetitively every 12 hr. (Fig. 11.1, Hint: There is an easy way to calculate the answer for the "ideal" tablet.) For each preparation suggest a dose and dose interval. (Chapters 10 & 11). Qualitatively, how would the concentrations differ if the clearance were doubled or halved with no change in the volume of distribution? How would this affect the suggested dosing schedule?

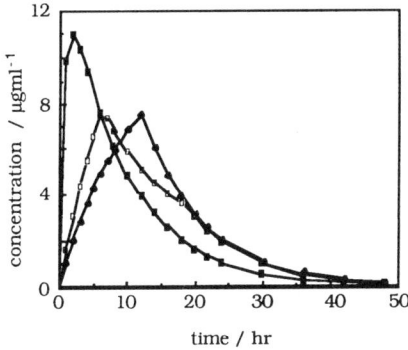

Figure E.1 Theophylline plasma concentrations following a 400 mg dose given as a conventional tablet (filled squares), as Uniphyllin Continus® (open squares), or as an "ideal" tablet (filled circles). Data from Table E.6

Table E.6 Plasma concentrations measured after 400 mg doses of theophylline

Time / hr	Concentration / $\mu g\,ml^{-1}$		
	Conventional dose	Uniphyllin Continus®	"Ideal tablet"
0	0.0	0.0	0.0
1	9.8	1.6	1.1
2	11.0	3.1	2.0
3	10.4	4.4	2.9
4	9.4	5.5	3.6
5		6.6	4.3
6	7.6	7.5	4.9
7		7.3	5.5
8	6.1	6.8	6.0
10	4.9	5.9	6.8
12	3.9	5.1	7.5
14	3.2	4.5	6.1
16	2.6	4.1	4.9
18	2.1	3.7	3.9
20	1.7	3.1	3.2
22	1.3	2.5	2.6
24	1.1	2.0	2.1
30	0.6	1.0	1.1
36	0.3	0.5	0.6
42	0.2	0.3	0.3
48	0.1	0.1	0.2

The experimental data for the conventional tablet and the Uniphyllin Continus® tablet are taken from A. Rhodes & S.T. Leslie (1984), in *New Perspectives in Theophylline Therapy*, Eds. M.Turner-Warwick. & J. Levy, Royal Society of Medicine International Congress and Symposium Series No. 78, Royal Society of Medicine, London, pp. 273-81. The "ideal" tablet releases theophylline at a constant rate for 12 hr. The plasma concentrations for the "ideal" tablet have been simulated using a beaker model with the clearance and rate constant for elimination calculated from the data for the conventional dose.

(3) In qualitative terms what would the consequences be for dosing with Uniphyllin or the "ideal" tablet if the unabsorbed remnant of the dose were lost in the faeces after 8 hr? (Chapter 10) What would happen if the patient were to take 400 mg at 8 am and 10 pm instead of once every 12 hr? Is the "ideal" tablet actually ideal?

E.2.10-12 Cytotoxic agents used in the treatment of cancer

The objective when administering cytotoxic drugs is to kill as many neoplastic cells as possible without producing unacceptable or intolerable toxicity to the rest of the body. The limiting toxicity is often suppression of bone marrow leading in severe cases to aplastic anaemia, the failure to produce blood cells. While there are as yet few firm principles that can be applied to dose adjustment, several general observations can be made.

(1) Accurate administration of the doses is often easiest by intravenous infusion.

(2) Both the desired results and the toxic effects can be difficult to assess in time to act as a guide for dosing.

(3) The pharmacokinetics of the agents can vary markedly between patients and this variation is likely to be an important contributor to variations in response.

(4) Each individual dose must be small enough to avoid acute toxicity. Thus a dose which might not be tolerated if given as a single bolus, may be acceptable if given as an infusion lasting for several hours or if divided into several doses to be administered at intervals.

(5) For some agents the rate at which cells are damaged sufficiently that they will die appears to be proportional to the plasma concentration of the agent. This rate is also greater for cells that divide frequently possibly because there is then less time available for intracellular repair before new DNA must be synthesized. For this type of agent the number of cells damaged sufficiently in an interval of time will be proportional to the product of the rate and the length of the time interval. Because the rate is proportional to concentration, the number damaged is proportional to the area under the concentration versus time curve for the interval, and (see Fig. 2.1) the total number of cells damaged by a dose will be proportional to the total AUC. Thus measured AUC should correlate more closely than dose with the effects.

(6) For some other agents cell killing requires that a sufficient concentration be maintained for a sufficient period of time. This could arise if the agent must be present at a critical stage of the cell cycle. The objective of dose regimen design for these agents is to maintain a sufficient concentration of the agent for the maximum period consistent with tolerable toxicity.

(7) For other agents the relations between concentration and effect is unknown and dosage is scaled on the basis of body size, usually per unit surface area (see Chapter 2).

The three exercises that follow provide illustrations of some of these points. They also provide more data for practice calculations.

E.2.10 Methotrexate: prediction from bolus dose data, analytical versus numerical estimation of the area

Supplementary references:

Jolivet,J., Cowan,K.H., Curt,G.A., Clendeninn,N.J. & Chabner,B.A. (1983), The pharmacology and clinical use of methotrexate, *N.Engl.J.Med.*, **309**,1094-104.

Bleyer,W.A. (1978), The clinical pharmacology of methotrexate, *Cancer*, **41**,36-51

Methotrexate is a folate analogue used in cancer chemotherapy. After entry to cells via the transporter for folate, it binds strongly to and inhibits dihydrofolate reductase leading to depletion of fully reduced folate within the cell. This depletion and possibly other effects lead to the death of cells that attempt to pass through the S phase of the cell cycle. Effective toxicity thus requires that a sufficient concentration of methotrexate be achieved in the target cells and that this concentration be maintained until the damage to the cells is irreversible.

The minimum, sustained plasma concentration that is toxic to bone marrow, the epithelium of the gut and non-resistant tumour cells is about $2 \cdot 10^{-8}$ mol litre^{-1}. Unfortunately successful inhibition of dihydrofolate reductase in resistant cells may require plasma concentrations approaching 10^{-3} mol litre^{-1} for a number of hours. Normal cells can usually be expected to survive total dihydrofolate reductase inhibition for up to 42 hr

Table E.7 The plasma concentrations produced by a 10 mg (22 µmol) dose of
methotrexate

time	C	time	C
hr	µmol litre^{-1}	hr	µmol litre^{-1}
0.02	5.56	10.00	0.042
0.10	3.44	20.00	0.014
0.50	1.24	30.00	0.0054
1.00	0.91	40.00	0.0020
2.00	0.54	50.00	0.0007
5.00	0.14		

Data taken from J. Edelman, D.F. Biggs, F. Jamali & A.S. Russell (1984), Low-dose
methotrexate kinetics in arthritis, *Clin.Pharmacol.Ther.* ,**35**,382-6.

provided a source of reduced folate then becomes available. The source can be either via
renewed activity of dihydrofolate reductase or "rescue treatment" using leucovorin.

(1) The plasma concentrations of methotrexate following a single 10 mg bolus dose are given
in Table E.7. Calculate the clearance, the terminal phase half-life, the initial volume of
distribution and the terminal phase volume of distribution. (Supplementary exercise:
calculate the steady-state volume of distribution.) (Fig. 2.2, Fig. 8.1 and Fig. S4.1).

(2) What bolus dose would be required to produce a concentration of 10^{-3} mol litre^{-1} at 10 hr?
When would the concentration fall below $2 \cdot 10^{-8}$ mol litre^{-1}? (Section 8.3).

(3) What infusion rate is required to maintain a concentration of 10^{-3} mol litre^{-1}? (Section
2.1). Calculate the concentration at the end of a 6 hr infusion at this rate. (Sections 9.1
and S4.3).

In one recommended dose schedule methotrexate is infused at 2.5 g hr^{-1}. The infusion is
stopped after 6 hr and a course of leucovorin once each 6 hr is begun. At 24 hr a blood sample
is taken, and the methotrexate concentration is used to adjust the leucovorin dose rate to
provide adequate rescue. Leucovorin must be continued until the methotrexate concentration
falls sufficiently to remove the inhibition of dihydrofolate reductase.

(4) If the plasma concentration in the 24 hr sample is $2 \cdot 10^{-5}$ mol litre^{-1}, how long will it take
for the concentration to fall below $2 \cdot 10^{-8}$ mol litre^{-1}? (Section 8.3).

E.2.11 Doxorubicin: dose escalation in phase one clinical trials

Supplementary reference:

Collins,J.M., Zaharko,D.S., Dedrick,R.L. & Chabner,B.A. (1986), Potential roles for
preclinical pharmacology in phase 1 clinical trials, *Cancer Treat. Rep.* ,**70**,73-80.

Doxorubicin (Adriamycin$^{®}$) is a cytotoxic drug whose main mechanism of action is to
interfere with nucleic acid metabolism by intercalating into DNA. As with many cytotoxic
agents, both the kill of neoplastic cells and the toxic effects are closely related to the product
of the plasma concentration and the time for which it is maintained, in other words to the
area under the curve, AUC. This suggests that the AUC for a test dose could be used to guide
subsequent treatment.

It has been observed that the maximum tolerated (cumulative) dose, MTD, for humans is
often close to the dose that kills 10% of test mice, LD_{10}, provided the doses are expressed per
unit surface area of the patient and the mouse respectively. However, even with this scaling
there is still a tenfold range of values for the ratio, MTD/LD_{10} when the data are inspected for
many drugs. In phase 1 clinical trials of new cytotoxic agents it is necessary to choose a safe
initial dose as well as a procedure for increasing the dose until toxicity is observed. The
increases must be small enough for the first observed toxicity to be mild, yet large enough to
reach therapeutic levels (if they exist) as quickly as possible. Thus when the dose is expected to
be far from toxic levels it should be increased rapidly, but as the MTD is approached the
increases should be smaller. One common practice is to start with one-tenth of the LD_{10} for
mice and to increase the doses according to a modified Fibonacci series until toxicity is
noted. In this series the dose is increased by the following steps: 100%, 50%, and 40%
followed by increases of 33%. If MTD <=LD_{10}, the MTD will be found within five or six steps.
However, when MTD > LD_{10} many steps can be required and no benefit is available over a
number of courses of treatment.

If effect were accurately proportional to AUC, the MTD could be predicted as

$$\text{predicted MTD} = \left(\frac{\text{AUC}_{\text{mouse}}}{\text{AUC}_{\text{test}}}\right)(\text{test dose})$$

However, a single large step from a test dose near $LD_{10}/10$ to the brink of toxicity is too risky. Two compromises have been proposed. In one, the first stage of escalation uses the geometric mean

$$\text{First stage dose} = \sqrt{(\text{predicted MTD})(\text{test dose})}$$

followed by the modified Fibonacci series (starting with a 100% increase). In the second proposal the dose is increased in steps of 100% up to 40% of the predicted MTD, and the escalation is then continued using the Fibonacci series starting with a 50% increase.

To ensure that these procedures would not have introduced additional risk, they have been applied retrospectively to a number of agents that have undergone phase 1 testing. For doxorubicin MTD/LD_{10} is 5 and the ratio of the AUC's in man at the MTD and in the mouse at the LD_{10} is

$$\frac{\text{AUC}_{\text{human MTD}}}{\text{AUC}_{\text{mouse } LD_{10}}} = 0.8$$

Calculate the number of escalation steps required by each of the three procedures discussed above.

E.2.12 Carboplatin : renal and systemic clearance; dose adjustment

Supplementary References:

Calvert,A.H., Newell,D.R., Gumbrell,L.A., O'Reilly,S., Burnell,M., Boxall,F.E., Siddik,Z.H., Judson,I.R., Gore,M.E. & Wiltshaw,E. (1989), Carboplatin dosage: prospective evaluation of a simple formula based on renal function, *J.Clin.Oncol.* ,**7**,1748-56.

Newell,D.R., Siddik,Z.H., Gumbrell,L.A., Boxall,F.E., Gore,M.E., Smith,I.E. & Calvert,A.H. (1987), Plasma free platinum pharmacokinetics in patients treated with high dose carboplatin, *Eur.J.Cancer Clin.Oncol.* ,**23**,1399-405.

Harland,S.J., Newell,D.R., Siddik,Z.H., Chadwick,R., Calvert,A.H. & Harrap,K.R. (1984), Pharmacokinetics of *cis*-diamine-1,1-cyclobutane dicarboxylate platinum(II) in patients with normal and impaired renal function, *Cancer Research* ,**44**,1693-7.

Egorin,M.J., van Echo,D.A., Tipping,S.J., Olman,E.A., Whitacre,M.Y., Thompson,B.W. & Aisner,J. (1984), Pharmacokinetics and dosage reduction of *cis*-diamine(1,1-cyclobutanedicarboxylato)platinum in patients with impaired renal function, *Cancer Research* ,**44**,5432-8.

Cisplatin is a platinum containing compound with cytotoxic activity against several types of tumours. However, its use and particularly its reuse have been severely restricted by cumulative damage to the kidneys and the inner ears. Carboplatin is a derivative of cisplatin that appears to be devoid of both these adverse affects. Its limiting toxicity is bone marrow depression producing a marked fall in the number of platelets in the blood and, to a lesser extent, a decrease in the white blood cell count. These toxicities are still dangerous in that total suppression is irreversible. Even when suppression is less marked and reversible, the patient's resistance to haemorrhage and infection can be severely impaired until bone marrow function recovers. Nevertheless with careful dose adjustment substantial selective toxicity to tumours has been achieved and, with intervals to allow the bone marrow to recover, repetitive treatment is possible.

The pharmacokinetics of carboplatin have been investigated extensively. In one such study, following a dose of 1.87 mmol carboplatin (MW 371), the total plasma concentration of platinum (regardless of the compounds of which it was part) was measured with the results given in the second column of Table E.8. The reason for the final slow stage was investigated further by preparing a protein free ultrafiltrate of plasma. The total concentration of platinum in this ultrafiltrate is given in the third column. In 24 hr 65% of the total amount of platinum was excreted by the kidneys (probably almost entirely as unchanged carboplatin). Virtually none could be found in the faeces.

(1) What are the values of the systemic or total clearance, the renal clearance, the half-life and the terminal phase volume of distribution? (Sections 2.3, 2.5, 8.2 and 8.5.2). Assuming that the 35% not accounted for in the urine is still in the body in what form is it likely to be found? What fraction is bound to the plasma proteins?

(2) Discuss the fate of free carboplatin. Assuming that the 35% not accounted for in the urine is still in the body in what form is it likely to be found? What fraction is bound to the plasma proteins? How does this binding differ from the binding to plasma proteins seen with most drugs?

In the initial trials it was observed that the onset of toxicity for patients occurred over a wide range of values for the total dose (expressed in mg m^{-2}). Furthermore the maximum tolerated dose was smaller in patients known to have partial renal failure. In a subsequent study the percentage reduction in platelet count (at the nadir) was found to correlate strongly with the area under the curve for free platinum versus time after a bolus dose.

(3) Suggest a basis for dose adjustment.

Table E.8 Plasma concentration following a 1.87 mmol dose of carboplatin

time	total platinum	free platinum
hr	µmol litre^{-1}	µmol litre^{-1}
0	61.4	61.40
1	42.7	42.17
2	30.3	29.38
3	21.9	20.79
4	16.3	14.94
5	12.4	10.90
6	9.6	8.07
8	6.3	4.61
10	4.5	2.75
15	2.7	0.86
20	2.2	0.29
25	2.0	0.10

E.3 ANSWERS

E.3.1   Lithium

(1) The half-life or equivalently the terminal phase rate constant is determined from a log plot, $\lambda_z = 0.023\,hr^{-1}$, $t_{1/2,z} = 20\,hr$. Assuming the availability is 1 the total clearance is calculated from the AUC for the plasma concentration data. This area may be calculated purely numerically or more conveniently by first drawing a log plot, determining $C_Z = 0.40\,mmol\,litre^{-1}$ and $\lambda_z = 0.023\,hr^{-1}$, and calculating the area under most of the curve as

$$AUC_{sc} = \frac{C_Z}{\lambda_z} = \frac{0.40\,mmol\,litre^{-1}}{0.023\,hr^{-1}} = 17.4\,mmol\,hr\,litre^{-1}.$$

The rest of the area above the single exponential but below the curve is estimated numerically and is approximately $3\,mmol\,hr\,litre^{-1}$. Thus

$$CL = \frac{D}{AUC} = \frac{20.3\,mmol}{20.4\,mmol\,hr\,litre^{-1}} = 1\,litre\,hr^{-1}.$$

The renal clearance is calculated as (rate of excretion)/ (plasma concentration). The rate of excretion from the table should be divided by the average plasma concentration during the dose interval. Provided that the intervals are short enough this will be approximately the concentration at the middle of the interval which is most simply determined from the log plot of the data. The renal clearance is also 1 litre hr^{-1}. The dose rate to achieve $1\,mmol\,litre^{-1}$ is $1\,mmol\,hr^{-1}$ which is $24\,mmol\,day^{-1}$.

2) The concentration just after a dose reflects the vagaries of the absorption process and is therefore not suitable for monitoring (see also the exercise for gentamicin). For a single measurement of the plasma concentration to reflect the actual value of the average concentration it should be taken near the middle of the dose interval. However, if all that is required is a standard value that can be used with a nomogram or rule of thumb, it is more convenient (at least with in-patients) to collect the sample just before a dose on the standard 12 hr cycle even though this concentration will be less than the average by an amount that varies with the half-life.

3) By ratio and proportion if $20.3\,mg$ doses produce $1.5\,mmol\,litre^{-1}$ and the target is $0.6\,mmol\,litre^{-1}$, the adjusted dose should be $20.3 \cdot 0.6 / 1.5 = 8\,mmol\,litre^{-1}$.

E.3.2 Digoxin

The single-compartment model provides an adequate description for oral doses of digoxin, because absorption is rapid compared to elimination and the terminal phase is reached before an appreciable fraction of a dose has been eliminated.

(1a) **Dose interval** (Section 11.3) Using a beaker model the maximum dose interval is

$$\tau_{max} = (t_{1/2,z} / 0.3)\,\log\,(C_{max}/C_{min})$$

The expected half-life may be calculated from the creatinine clearance,

$$t_{1/2} = 110\,hr / (1 + 1.2 \cdot 1.45) = 40\,hr$$

and thus

$$\tau_{max} = (40\,hr /0.3)\,\log(1.8/1) = 34\,hr$$

In practice either 12 hr or 24 hr is chosen so that the dose interval will be easy to remember.

(1b) **Dose** The dose may be estimated from the pharmacokinetic constants and a target average concentration (see Section 11.1). For dose intervals shorter than a half-life the average concentration is approximately half-way between C_{max} and C_{min}, i.e. $1.4\,ng\,ml^{-1}$, and the dose rate to produce this average concentration may be calculated as

$$D = DR \cdot \tau = \frac{C_{av,ss} \cdot CL \cdot \tau}{F}$$

Thus for $\tau = 24\,hr$ and using

$$CL = (0.88 \cdot 1.45 + 0.33)\,ml\,min^{-1}\,kg^{-1} \cdot 70\,kg = 112\,ml\,min^{-1}$$

$$D = \frac{1.4 \, \text{ng ml}^{-1} \cdot 10^{-3} \, \mu\text{g ng}^{-1} \cdot 112 \, \text{ml min}^{-1} \cdot 24 \text{hr} \cdot 60 \, \text{min hr}^{-1}}{0.7} = 322 \, \mu\text{g}$$

The practical choice is between $312.5 \, \mu\text{g day}^{-1}$ and $375 \, \mu\text{g day}^{-1}$. With either choice the outcome should be reviewed and the dosage adjusted subsequently. (The dose can also be calculated as outlined in Fig. 11.3.)

(2) **Predicted maximum and minimum concentrations after each dose.** The beaker volume is calculated as

$$V_z = \frac{CL}{\lambda_z} = CL \cdot t_{1/2} / 0.69$$

$$= \frac{112 \, \text{ml min}^{-1} \cdot 10^{-3} \, \text{litre ml}^{-1} \cdot 40 \text{hr} \cdot 60 \, \text{min hr}^{-1}}{0.69} = 390 \, \text{litre}$$

and the concentration after each dose increases by (see Fig. 11.3)

$$C_0 = \frac{D \cdot F}{V_z} = \frac{375 \, \mu\text{g} \cdot 10^3 \, \text{ng} \, \mu\text{g}^{-1} \cdot 0.7}{390 \, \text{litre} \cdot 10^3 \, \text{ml litre}^{-1}} = 0.67 \, \text{ng ml}^{-1}.$$

The calculation can now proceed by either of the routes indicated in Figs. 11.1 and 11.3. After a single dose the concentration decreases exponentially following

$$C = C_{i,max} \, e^{-\lambda_z t} = C_{i,max} \, e^{-0.69 \cdot t / t_{1,2}}$$

Thus after one dose interval τ,

$$C_{i,min} = C_{i,max} \, e^{-0.69 \cdot \tau / t_{1,2}} = C_{i,max} \, e^{-0.69 \cdot 24 \text{hr} / 40 \text{hr}} = C_{i,max} \cdot 0.66$$

Following the procedure of Fig. 11.3, the concentrations after each dose are

Dose	$C_{i,max}/(\text{ng ml}^{-1})$	$C_{i,min}/(\text{ng ml}^{-1})$
First	0.67	$0.67 \cdot 0.66 = 0.44$
Second	$0.44 + 0.67 = 1.11$	$1.11 \cdot 0.66 = 0.73$
Third	$0.73 + 0.67 = 1.40$	$1.40 \cdot 0.66 = 0.93$
Fourth	$0.93 + 0.67 = 1.60$	$1.60 \cdot 0.66 = 1.05$
Fifth	$1.05 + 0.67 = 1.72$	$1.72 \cdot 0.66 = 1.14$
	etc.	

After many doses this sequence must start repeating itself, i.e.

$$C_{max} = C_{min} + 0.67 \, \text{ng ml}^{-1} \qquad \text{and} \qquad C_{min} = C_{max} \cdot 0.66$$

must both be satisfied at the same time which leads to

$$C_{max} = C_{max} \cdot 0.66 + 0.67 = 0.67 / (1 - 0.66) = 1.97 \, \text{ng ml}^{-1}$$

$$C_{min} = 1.3 \, \text{ng ml}^{-1}$$

The alternative method in Fig. 11.1 is more general in that it can be used even when the concentration does not vary exponentially with time. Of course, when the concentration does vary exponentially it gives the same answers. For instance using c(t) to represent the concentration after a single dose, C_{max} after four doses is

$$C_{4,max} = c(0) + c(24 \, \text{hr}) + c(48 \, \text{hr}) + c(72 \, \text{hr}) = 0.67 \, \text{ng ml}^{-1} \cdot (1 + 0.66 + 0.66^2 + 0.66^3) = 1.6 \, \text{ng ml}^{-1}$$

The minimum concentration after the third dose is just this value minus $0.67 \, \text{ng ml}^{-1}$.

By either route of calculation the concentration first exceeds $1 \, \text{ng ml}^{-1}$ on the second day. It last falls below that level on the third. There are two important consequences. Firstly, if treatment is started with the maintenance dose, full effects will be produced only after a considerable delay. Secondly these effects can not be assessed for many days. For instance if toxicity were to appear at $1.8 \, \text{ng ml}^{-1}$ this would only become apparent after six or more days of treatment.

(3) **Loading dose** (Section 11.5). Use either ratio and proportion

$$\frac{C_{max}}{\text{Loading Dose}} = \frac{C_0}{\text{Maintenance Dose}}$$

or

$$\text{Loading Dose} = AR \cdot D = \frac{D}{\left(\begin{array}{c}\text{fraction of a dose lost}\\ \text{in the first dose interval}\end{array}\right)}$$

where (Fig. 11.3)

$$AR = \frac{1}{1 - e^{-0.69 \cdot \tau / t_{1/2}}} = \frac{1}{1 - e^{-0.69 \cdot 24hr/40hr}} = 2.94$$

Thus

$$\text{Loading Dose} = 312.5 \, \mu g \cdot 2.94 = 920 \, \mu g$$

For safety it is standard practice to give the loading dose divided into three or more parts with time allowed for each to develop its full effects. If toxic effects are noted subsequent doses are reduced. A satisfactory procedure was stated in part 4 of the question.

(4) The **loading dose** and the **maintenance dose** are related by (see Sections 11.2 and 11.5)

$$D = \text{Loading dose} \cdot \left\{ \begin{array}{c}\text{fraction of the loading dose}\\ \text{lost during the dose interval}\end{array} \right\}$$

From the preceding section

$$\text{fraction lost} = 1 - e^{-0.69 \cdot \tau / t_{1/2}} = 1 - e^{-0.69 \cdot 24hr/40hr} = \frac{1}{AR} = 0.34$$

and the predicted maintenance dose is $1250 \, \mu g \cdot 0.34 = 425 \, \mu g$.

If instead the creatinine clearance is $0.5 \, ml \, min^{-1} \, kg^{-1}$,

$$\text{fraction lost} = 1 - e^{-0.69 \cdot 24hr/69hr} = 1 - 0.79 = 0.21$$

and the maintenance dose would then be only $1250 \, \mu g \cdot 0.21 = 263 \, \mu g$.

This calculation can be made particularly simple by noting that the relations between the fraction lost, the half-life, and the creatinine clearance can be combined to yield

$$\text{fraction lost per day} = 0.14(1 + CL_{Cr}) \text{ for } CL_{Cr} \text{ in ml min}^{-1} \, kg^{-1}$$

or

$$\text{percentage lost per day} = 14 + CL_{Cr}/5 \text{ for } CL_{Cr} \text{ in ml min}^{-1}$$

E.3.3 Lignocaine

The infusion rate required to maintain a steady-state concentration of $2.65 \, \mu g \, ml^{-1}$ is

$$R_0 = CL \cdot C_{ss} = 650 \, ml \, min^{-1} \cdot 2.65 \, \mu g \, ml^{-1} = 1.7 \, mg \, min^{-1}$$

while the loading dose predicted for a beaker with $V_{beaker} = V_z$ is

$$\text{Loading dose} = C_{ss} \cdot V_{beaker} = C_{ss} \frac{CL \cdot t_{1/2}}{0.69}$$

$$= 2.65 \, \mu g \, ml^{-1} \frac{650 \, ml \, min^{-1} \cdot 110 \, min}{0.69} = 275 \, mg$$

The concentration in a beaker following the bolus dose follows

$$C = C_{ss} e^{-k_{el}t}$$

while the concentration after the start of the infusion follows

$$C = C_{ss} (1 - e^{-k_{el}t})$$

where $k_{el} = 0.69/t_{1/2}$. When these concentrations are added together, the resulting concentration remains constant at C_{ss} for all times after the initial loading dose. Thus a beaker or single-compartment model predicts that the concentration can be controlled by the combination of a single bolus dose and a constant infusion. **This prediction is wrong and the bolus loading dose calculated from it may be dangerously large.** The predicted time course for the infusion is reasonable (see Section S4.3), but the concentrations following a bolus dose do not follow a single-exponential. When the dose is first given most is taken to the tissues with high blood flow and the concentrations in these tissues and in plasma are much higher than in other parts of the body. The actual plasma concentration would start some threefold higher than predicted by the beaker model and would then decrease over about an hour towards the steady-state level. A reliable method of calculation is described in Chapter 9 (the equations are stated in Section S4.3). The loading dose, calculated as $C_{ss}V_{ss}$ which is about two-thirds of $C_{ss}V_z$, is divided into an initial bolus of about $(1/2) \cdot C_{ss}V_{ss}$ followed by infusion at a rate greater than needed for steady-state maintenance until loading is nearly complete.

E.3.4   Gentamicin

The terminal phase for gentamicin can be described as

$$C = \frac{D}{V_{app}} e^{-\lambda_z t}$$

where V_{app} is a proportionality constant. If the body were a beaker, it would be the volume of distribution. The terminal phase rate constant can be calculated using

$$\frac{C(1hr)}{C(8hr)} = \frac{e^{-1hr \cdot \lambda_z}}{e^{-8hr \cdot \lambda_z}} = e^{-7hr \cdot \lambda_z}$$

$$\lambda_z = 0.125 \, hr^{-1}$$

For a target trough concentration of $1.5 \, \mu g \, ml^{-1}$ and a target peak:of gentamicin of $7.5 \, \mu g \, ml^{-1}$ the interval between the samples, T-1, should be a bit more than two half-lives,

$$T = 1 + \frac{1}{\lambda_z} \ln\frac{7.5}{1.5} = 13.9 \, hr$$

In practice a dose interval of 12hr would be used with the dose adjusted for a lower peak sample concentration

$$C(1hr) = \frac{C(12 \, hr)}{e^{-\lambda_z \cdot 11 \, hr}} = \frac{1.5 \, \mu g \, ml^{-1}}{0.253} = 5.9 \, \mu g \, ml^{-1}$$

Following a dose at steady-state, the concentration is to increase from $1.5 \, \mu g \, ml^{-1}$ to its true peak from which it will fall somewhat before the sample at 1hr. During this hour the concentration resulting from all previous doses will continue to fall exponentially decreasing from $1.5 \, \mu g \, ml^{-1}$ to $1.5 \, \mu g \, ml^{-1} \cdot e^{-\lambda_z \cdot 1 \, hr} = 1.3 \, \mu g \, ml^{-1}$. The dose must make up the difference between this tail resulting from all previous doses and the target values, i.e it must produce a concentration after 1 hr equal to $5.9 - 1.3 = 4.6 \mu g \, ml^{-1}$. By ratio and proportion since $1.5 \, mg \, kg^{-1}$ produced $12 \, \mu g \, ml^{-1}$, the dose required is $(4.6/12) \cdot 1.5 = 0.58 \, mg \, kg^{-1}$.

E.3.5   Phenytoin

(1) Because the rate of elimination of phenytoin is not proportional to its plasma concentration, it is not correct to use the equations for multiple dosing presented in Chapter 11. However, for there to be a steady state it is still necessary that

average rate of elimination = average rate of absorption

As a first guess assume that the concentration remains constant at an average value, C_1. Then

$$\text{rate of elimination} = \frac{7.5 \, mg \, kg^{-1} \, day^{-1} \cdot C_1}{C_1 + 5.7 \, \mu g \, ml^{-1}} = \frac{300 \, mg \, day^{-1}}{50 \, kg} = 6 \, mg \, kg^{-1} \, day^{-1}$$

which implies

$$C_1 = 22.8 \, \mu g \, ml^{-1}$$

To estimate the variation in concentration calculate the amount of phenytoin in the body and the change in this amount which occurs after each dose. The average amount is $22.8 \, \mu g \, ml^{-1} \cdot 0.64 \, litre \, kg^{-1} \cdot 50 \, kg \cdot 1000 \, ml \, litre^{-1} = 730 \, mg$. Thus each dose produces a change in amount which is roughly $(100/730) \cdot 100 = 14\%$ of the average. This is a small variation, and therefore the average concentration will be very near the middle of the range and a reasonable approximation would be to say that the concentration varies between $22.8 + 0.07 \cdot 22.8 \,\mu g\,ml^{-1} = 24.4 \,\mu g\,ml^{-1}$ and $22.8 - 0.07 \cdot 22.8 \,\mu g\,ml^{-1} = 21.2 \,\mu g\,ml^{-1}$. There is little point, but the estimates can be refined further by calculating the amount eliminated as the concentration falls from its maximum to its minimum and then refining the limits so that both the amount eliminated in each dose interval and the increase in concentration produced by each dose are correct.

(2) The dose rate for $C = 45.6 \,\mu g\,ml^{-1}$ is

$$\frac{7.5\,mg\,kg^{-1}\,day^{-1} \cdot 45.6 \mu gml^{-1}}{45.6 \,\mu g\,ml^{-1} + 5.7\,\mu g\,ml^{-1}} = 6.67\,mg\,kg^{-1}\,day^{-1}$$

Thus an eleven per cent increase in dose rate produces a doubling of the steady-state concentration. Dosage must be adjustable in small increments.

(3) The 25% increase from $6\,mg\,kg^{-1}\,day^{-1}$ to $7.5\,mg\,kg^{-1}\,day^{-1}$ will eventually lead to an infinite increase in concentration, that is a concentration that continues to increase in time without limit. The extra dose of $75\,mg\,day^{-1}$ can at most increase the concentration by $75\,mg\,day^{-1}/V_z$ which expressed as a percentage of the existing plasma concentration is $100 \cdot$ (amount added)/(amount present) $= 100 \cdot 75/730 = 10\%$. Thus the concentration will take at least 10 days to double. There are two important consequences. Firstly monitoring must be extended for many days to detect the consequences of any change. Secondly, while errors in dose rate can have very serious consequences, the changes in plasma concentration occur slowly enough that they can be detected by routine plasma concentration monitoring before adverse effects occur.

(4) Enzyme induction will increase the rate of elimination of phenytoin which can produce a large decrease in its plasma concentration. The effects of this decrease may be masked by the effects produced by the second agent.

(5) For the new maximum rate of elimination, $7.0\,mg\,kg^{-1}\,day^{-1}$, the concentration must satisfy

$$\frac{7.0\,mg\,kg^{-1}\,day^{-1} \cdot C}{C + 5.7\,\mu g\,ml^{-1}} = 6\,mg\,kg^{-1}\,day^{-1}$$

$$C = 34\,\mu g\,ml^{-1}$$

To restore the original concentration the dose rate must be reduced in proportion to the change in the maximum rate of elimination, i.e. to $6 \cdot (7/7.5) = 5.6\,mg\,kg^{-1}\,day^{-1}$.

E.3.6 Dicloxacillin

The clearance and all three volumes of distribution are smaller for dicloxacillin. These changes are a result of substantially increased binding to plasma proteins. Thus following a dose, a larger fraction remains in the plasma initially, so that $V_{initial}$ is smaller. At steady state for a given plasma concentration, the free concentration and hence the amount in the tissues will be smaller and V_{ss} will be reduced. The clearance is smaller because the reduction in the free concentration reduces the rate of secretion into the proximal tubules. Even for the other penicillins secretion is not so fast that it could produce complete extraction of the drug from plasma. Smaller clearance means that V_z will be closer to V_{ss} for dicloxacillin than the others. The effects of plasma protein binding on the pharmacokinetic constants is considered more fully in Supplement 2.

E.3.7 Warfarin

(1) The dose rate required to produce $1.2 \,\mu g\,ml^{-1}$ is $DR = CL \cdot 1.2 \,\mu g\,ml^{-1} = 5.2\,mg\,day^{-1}$. Because the half-life is long, once daily dosing is adequate. Thus the expected dose is near $5\,mg$ given once daily.

(2) The volume of the beaker is

$$V_z = \frac{CL \cdot t_{1/2}}{0.69} = \frac{180\,ml\,hr^{-1} \cdot 37\,hr}{0.69} = 9.7\,litre,$$

and the increase in concentration for each 5 mg dose is $0.51 \, \mu g \, ml^{-1}$. In a dose interval the concentration falls exponentially such that at the end

$$C_{end} = C_{start} \, e^{-\lambda_z t} = C_{start} \, e^{-24hr \cdot 0.69/37 \, hr} = C_{start} \, 0.64$$

Letting c(t) represent the concentration following a single dose, the concentrations after the first few doses are (see Fig. 11.1) :

$C_{max,1}$	$= c(0)$	$= 0.51 \, \mu g \, ml^{-1}$	
$C_{max,2}$	$= c(0) + c(24 \, hr)$	$= 0.51 \, \mu g \, ml^{-1}(1 + 0.64)$	$= 0.84 \, \mu g \, ml^{-1}$
$C_{max,3}$	$= c(0) + c(24 \, hr) + c(48 \, hr)$	$= 0.51 \, \mu g \, ml^{-1}(1 + 0.64 + 0.64^2)$	$= 1.05 \, \mu g \, ml^{-1}$

Thus $1 \, \mu g \, ml^{-1}$ is exceeded after the third dose..

The dose interval is less than the half-life for warfarin. Thus the average concentration will be approximately half-way between the maximum and minimum concentrations for the interval, i.e.

$$C_{av,i} \approx C_{max,i} (1 + 0.64)/2 \quad = 0.82 \cdot C_{max,i} \, .$$

Continuing the series:

$C_{av,3} = 1.05 \, \mu g \, ml^{-1} \cdot 0.82 = 0.86 \, \mu g \, ml^{-1}$

$C_{av,4} = 0.97 \, \mu g \, ml^{-1}$

$C_{av,5} = 1.06 \, \mu g \, ml^{-1}$

The important point is that it takes a long time.

(3) The time at which the concentration of warfarin falls to $1.2 \, \mu g \, ml^{-1}$ can be estimated by solving

$$\frac{D}{V_{beaker}} \, e^{-\lambda_z t} = \frac{75 \, mg}{9.7 \, litre} \, e^{-0.69 \cdot t/37 \, hr} = 1.2 \, \mu g \, ml^{-1}$$

with the result $t = 100 \, hr$. If synthesis were to remain completely inhibited for this period, the clotting factor activity would fall to

$$100\% \cdot e^{-k_{deg} t} = 100\% \cdot e^{-(0.69 \cdot 100 \, hr/20 \, hr)} = 100\% \cdot 0.032 = 3.2\%$$

(4) Following a reduction in the rate of synthesis, clotting factor activity will decrease towards its new steady value. The quantity which decreases exponentially (see Chapter 9) is the difference between the present activity, Act, and the final value, Act_{ss}, i.e.

$$Act - Act_{ss} = (Act_{initial} - Act_{ss}) \, e^{-0.69 \cdot t/t_{1/2,deg}}$$

Thus when the starting point is 100% and the final 0%, the activity after 24hr would be

$$Act = Act_{initial} e^{-0.69 \cdot t/t_{1/2,deg}}$$

$$= 100\% \cdot 0.44 = 44\%$$

while for an average level of inhibition of 90%, $Act_{ss} = 10\%$ and

$$Act = 10\% + 90\% \cdot 0.44 = 50\%$$

The decrease in activity is larger after total inhibition, 56% versus 50%, but not much. Total inhibition is not required for the initial reduction in activity.

(5) If the starting point is 40% activity, the time for activity to decrease to 25% can be calculated from the equation used in part 5. Thus for 90% inhibition of synthesis

$$Act - Act_{ss} = (Act_{initial} - Act_{ss}) \, e^{-0.69 \cdot t/t_{1/2,deg}}$$

$$t = \frac{t_{1/2,deg}}{0.69} \ln \left[\frac{Act_{initial} - Act_{ss}}{Act - Act_{ss}} \right]$$

$$t = \frac{20 \, hr}{0.69} \ln \left[\frac{40-10}{25-10} \right] = 20 \, hr$$

while for 80% inhibition

$$t = \frac{20\,hr}{0.69}\ ln[\frac{40-20}{25-20}] = 40\,hr$$

Thus the final approach to the target can be substantially faster if synthesis can be "overinhibited" for an appropriate period of time. The critical period of time is not day 1, but rather days 3 to 5. It is, of course, important to reduce the dose rate after day 3 (see below).

(6) The calculation proceeds as in part 2 or by the route indicated in Fig 11.3:

$C_{max,1}$ = 1.03 μg ml⁻¹ ;

$C_{min,1}$ = 1.03 μg ml⁻¹ · 0.64 = 0.66 μg ml⁻¹;

$C_{max,2}$ = 0.66 μg ml⁻¹ + 1.03 μg ml⁻¹ = 1.69 μg ml⁻¹; $C_{min,2}$ = 1.69 μg ml⁻¹ · 0.64 = 1.08 μg ml⁻¹;

$C_{max,3}$ = 1.08 μg ml⁻¹ + 1.03 μg ml⁻¹ = 2.11 μg ml⁻¹; $C_{min,3}$ = 2.11 μg ml⁻¹ · 0.64 = 1.35 μg ml⁻¹;

$C_{max,4}$ = 1.35 μg ml⁻¹ + 0.51 μg ml⁻¹ = 1.86 μg ml⁻¹; $C_{min,4}$ = 1.86 μg ml⁻¹ · 0.64 = 1.19 μg ml⁻¹;

$C_{max,5}$ = 1.19 μg ml⁻¹ + 0.51 μg ml⁻¹ = 1.70 μg ml⁻¹; $C_{min,5}$ = 1.70 μg ml⁻¹ · 0.64 =1.09 μg ml⁻¹;

$C_{max,5}$ = 1.09 μg ml⁻¹ + 0.51 μg ml⁻¹ = 1.60 μg ml⁻¹; $C_{min,5}$ = 1.60 μg ml⁻¹ · 0.64 =1.02 μg ml⁻¹.

Thus in a "typical" patient this procedure produces a slight excess of warfarin concentration from day 2 to roughly day 5 or 6. This excess will, by reducing the rate of synthesis below the steady-state level, lead to faster depletion of the clotting factor activity.

(7) The variability between patients requires dose adjustment which would be very time consuming without some form of loading procedure. The severity of the consequences of overanticoagulation in turn strongly recommends a procedure which can be modified in mid-course to avoid overdose. The procedure recommended by Fennerty et al. in which loading is carried out over a period of three days, sacrifices a small amount of speed to gain a large increase in safety compared to a single loading dose. By monitoring the INR after each dose and comparing the results with previous findings, it is possible to anticipate excessive anticoagulation before it occurs. An appreciable increase in the prothrombin time (INR > 1.8) 18 hr after the first dose implies that only a small second dose is required. Similarly INR > 2 18 hr after the second dose requires reduction of the third loading dose. The INR 18 hr after the third dose (given according to the recipe with any previous adjustments) shows an excellent correlation with the maintenance dose that will be required. For most patients three 10 mg doses are given.

E.3.8   Tricyclic antidepressants.

The actual reason remains unknown. There are at least five plausible sources of variability in the response to a fixed dose that would produce effects that do not correlate with the plasma concentrations that have been measured.

(1) **Changes in the fraction free.** The tricyclic antidepressants are eliminated by metabolism in the liver with an extraction ratio near one. Thus the rate of elimination is determined by the rate at which the drug is delivered to the liver regardless of whether it is free or bound (see Sections 5.2 and 5.4). It follows that the clearance and the total steady-state, average plasma concentration will not be affected by a change in the percentage bound. A change in the percentage bound at constant total concentration implies a change in the free concentration. As the effects should correlate with the free rather than with the total concentration, variations in the percentage bound are expected to produce variability in response not accompanied by changes in total concentration (see Supplement 2). This suggestion should be tested by direct measurement of the percentage bound in plasma. Two fold variations have been observed in healthy volunteers

(2) **Active metabolites.** The tricyclic antidepressants can be metabolized by more than one route. It is conceivable that metabolites whose concentrations were not measured (e.g. the known hydroxylated metabolites) account for the effects observed. Variability in response would then reflect variations in the rate and extent of production of particular metabolites rather than the concentration of the parent drug and/or the measured metabolites.

(3) **Variable penetration into the brain.** To exert their effects the tricyclic antidepressants must cross the blood-brain barrier. Even in the steady-state, CSF concentrations of poorly permeant drugs may fail to reach equilibrium with plasma (see Section 4.6). The tricyclics

themselves are highly lipid soluble and thus will penetrate quite rapidly such that the concentration in CSF will reach equilibrium with the free concentration in plasma. However, there may be concentration differences for more polar metabolites. None of the attempts to correlate effects with concentration have determined these CSF concentrations. Variations in the rate of penetration through the blood brain barrier could produce variability in response that fails to correlate with plasma concentration.

(4) **Variations in the type of depression.** Depression is not a single well defined clinical entity, and a significant number of patients fail to gain any benefit from the tricyclic antidepressants. A major element in the variability of the response may thus be that more than one type of disorder is being treated. These disorders may have different sensitivities to the changes induced by these drugs. A classification of patients into groups requiring high or low concentrations for response might lead to the discovery of other significant differences between them.

(5) **Pharmacodynamic variation.** Variability in response to a given free concentration at the site of action can reflect differences in the properties of these sites or the manner in which the immediate effects are coupled to the response being measured. For instance genetic variation in the properties of binding sites can change the affinity for a drug.

It would be wrong to conclude on the present evidence either that all patients should be treated using a fixed daily dose (the procedure outlined in the question is much better) or that there would be no benefit from knowing the concentration produced by a dose. A fixed dose is used in this type of study so that data for all patients will be comparable. However, the choice of the fixed dose to use must be a compromise, and inevitably it will leave important questions unanswered. Would responders with high concentrations respond to a lower dose? Would a fraction of non-responders with low concentrations respond to a higher dose? When dose has been adjusted for optimal effect, is the range of concentrations significantly less than the range of the doses? Depending on the answers to these questions, plasma concentration monitoring may still allow more rapid, safe adjustment of dosage.

E.3.9 Theophylline

(1) The rate constant for elimination and the half-life can be determined from a plot on semi-log paper or by taking logs and plotting the values on linear paper. For both sets of real data the answer is the same, $\lambda_z = 0.108 \, hr^{-1}$ or $t_{1/2.z} = 6.4 \, hr$. The area under the curve may be calculated using the data provided and a sequence of trapezoids (see Fig. 2.2). For all three curves the answer is $123 \, \mu g \, hr \, ml^{-1}$. Thus CL/F is $54 \, ml \, min^{-1}$. Because the clearance should be the same regardless of the formulation of the dose, these curves imply that the availability is the same for the two real dose forms.

The average concentrations for all three dose forms and for both the suggested schedules will be the same

$$C_{av} = \frac{DR}{CL} = \frac{400 \, mg}{720 \, min \cdot 54 \, ml \, min^{-1}} = 10.3 \, \mu g \, ml^{-1}$$

If the clearance were doubled the average concentration would be halved. Thus for the same effect the dose rate should be doubled. Similarly if the clearance is halved, the dose rate should be reduced in proportion.

(2)   The multi-dose curves can be constructed graphically or by arithmetic calculation. For instance, using c(t) to represent the data for a single controlled release dose, at $t=77 \, hr$ (see Fig. 11.1)

$$C(77 \, hr) = \quad c(77 \, hr) \; + c(65 \, hr) \; + c(53 \, hr) \; + c(41 \, hr) \; + c(29 \, hr) \; + c(17 \, hr) \; + \quad\quad c(5 \, hr)$$
$$= \quad \sim 0 + \quad \sim 0 + \quad 0.1 + \quad 0.3 + \quad 1.1 + \quad 3.9 + \quad 6.6$$
$$= \quad 12 \, \mu g \, ml^{-1}$$

Data for doses given more than about $48 \, hr$ earlier can be ignored because their concentrations have decreased to negligible proportions. The results of these calculations for the three preparations are displayed in Fig. E.2.

The variation between the maximum and minimum concentrations should be less than two-fold. For the conventional formulation $12 \, hr$ dosing has given three-fold. Thus an acceptable dose interval is expected to be either $6 \, hr$ or $8 \, hr$. The average concentration should

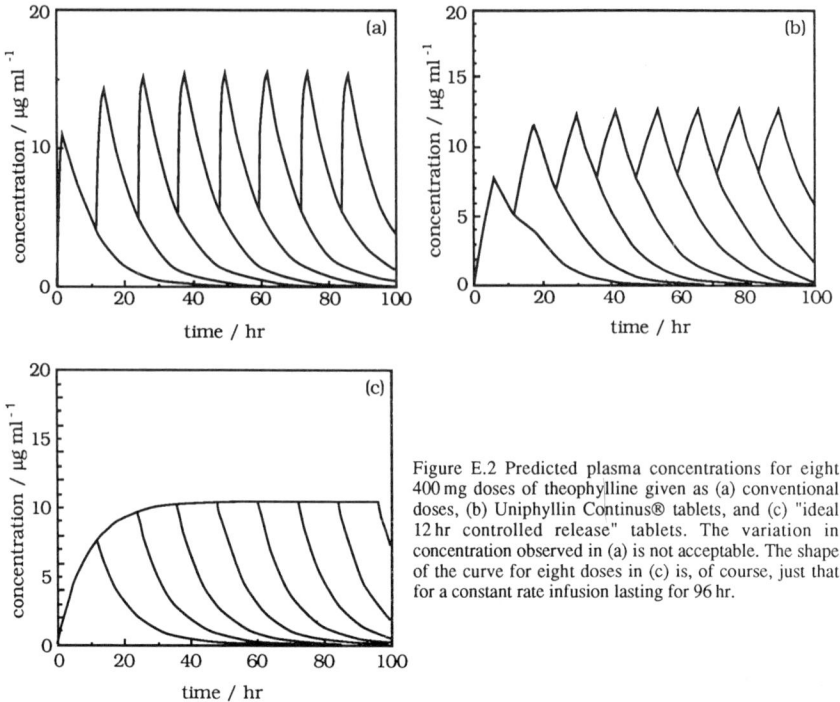

Figure E.2 Predicted plasma concentrations for eight 400 mg doses of theophylline given as (a) conventional doses, (b) Uniphyllin Continus® tablets, and (c) "ideal 12 hr controlled release" tablets. The variation in concentration observed in (a) is not acceptable. The shape of the curve for eight doses in (c) is, of course, just that for a constant rate infusion lasting for 96 hr.

be between $10 \mu g \, ml^{-1}$ and $15 \mu g \, ml^{-1}$ thus the dose rate should be about 600 mg/12 hr or, assuming an 8 hr interval and 125 mg tablets, probably 375 mg once each 8 hr. For Uniphyllin Continus® 12 hr dosing produces acceptable variation, and the expected dose size would be either 400 mg or 600 mg.

For both preparations doubled clearance requires the dose rate to be twice as large. Furthermore, if there is no change in the volume of distribution, the half-life for elimination will be approximately half as long. For the conventional preparation, the half-life for elimination is the half-life for the plasma concentration and the dose interval must be reduced to 3 hr to 4 hr. Such a short dose interval would be very inconvenient for chronic treatment. With the sustained release preparation plasma concentrations can be maintained for at least as long as absorption continues, and thus the required dose interval does not decrease in proportion to the change in the elimination half-life. It may be possible to maintain a dose interval of 12 hr.

If the clearance were half as large, for both preparations the dose rate would need to be halved. For the conventional preparation, 12 hr dosing would now be practical. For the sustained release preparation 12 hr dosing would still be optimal.

(3) From the shape of the concentration versus time curve for a single dose of Uniphyllin Continus® it is apparent that most of the dose is released in the first six hours. Thus premature passage of the remnant of the dose into the faeces after 8 hr will have little effect. For the "ideal 12 hr tablet" elimination of the remnant after 8 hr would decrease the availability to 0.67 which might lead to loss of effect.

The replacement of the 12 hr cycle by alternating 10 and 14 hr dose intervals (these can be constructed by superposition just as for the 12 hr cycle) results in slightly greater variation for Uniphyllin. For the "ideal" tablet the cycle is now 10 hr with the correct infusion rate, 2 hr with none, 10 hr correct, 2 hr double, 10 hr correct, etc. Two hours with no infusion can change the concentration by a factor of about $e^{-k_{el} \cdot 2 \, hr} = e^{-0.22} = 0.8$ while double the rate could increase it by about 1.2. These variations are comparable to those produced using Uniphyllin.

E.3.10 Methotrexate

1)The area under the curve may be calculated numerically or analytically. The numerical calculation is carried out via trapezoids in Table E.9 (see also Fig. 2.2). The alternative analytical calculation is based upon fitting a function to the data and then calculating the area under the curve using calculus. A triple exponential is fitted to the data in Fig. E.3 and Table E.10. The AUC is calculated from the peeled lines as

$$AUC = \frac{C_1}{\lambda_1} + \frac{C_2}{\lambda_2} + \frac{C_3}{\lambda_3}$$

$$= 4.06\,\mu mol\,hr\,litre^{-1}$$

The clearance is

$$CL = \frac{D}{AUC} = \frac{22\,\mu mol}{4.07\,\mu mol\,hr\,litre^{-1}} = 5.4\,litre\,hr^{-1}.$$

The terminal phase half-life is most easily obtained from the log plot (see Fig. E.3) and $\lambda_z = \lambda_3 = 7.1$ hr. The initial volume of distribution, $V_{initial} = 3.5$ litre^{-1} is calculated as dose divided by the extrapolated value of C at t=0, 6.4 $\mu mol\,litre^{-1}$. The terminal phase volume of distribution $V_z = 58$ litre^{-1} is calculated as CL/λ_z. The calculation of the steady-state volume of distribution is outlined in Fig. S3.2.

(2) The dose that would produce a concentration of 1 mmol litre^{-1} after 10 hr can be calculated by ratio and proportion from the concentration produced by the 10 mg (22 μmol) dose, i.e. D = $(10^{-3}\,mol\,litre^{-1}/4 \cdot 10^{-8}\,mol\,litre^{-1}) \cdot 10\,mg = 250$ g. It is not practical to give such a large dose. From Fig. E.3 the rate constant and intercept for the terminal phase after a dose of 10 mg are 0.1 $\mu mol\,litre^{-1}$ and 0.097 hr^{-1} respectively. The terminal phase for a dose of 250 gm would have an intercept of 2.5 mmol litre^{-1}. Thus the time at which the concentration will fall to

Table E.9 Calculation of the area under the curve using trapezoids. Concentrations measured after a 10 mg dose of methotrexate

Time hr	C $\mu mol\,litre^{-1}$	$\frac{C(i)+C(i-1)}{2}$ $\mu mol\,litre^{-1}$	Time interval	Area for interval
0.02	5.56	11.12	0.02	0.12
0.10	3.44	9.00	0.08	0.36
0.20	2.20	5.64	0.10	0.28
0.50	1.24	3.44	0.30	0.52
1.00	0.91	2.15	0.50	0.54
2.00	0.54	1.45	1.00	0.73
5.00	0.14	0.68	3.00	1.02
10.00	0.042	0.182	5.00	0.46
20.00	0.014	0.056	10.00	0.28
30.00	0.0054	0.019	10.00	0.095
40.00	0.0020	0.007	10.00	0.035
50.00	0.0007	0.002	10.00	0.015

The AUC is estimated as the sum of the areas for all of the data intervals, here 4.5 $\mu mol\,hr\,litre^{-1}$ (The area for the first interval has been estimated as a rectangle of height C(0.02 hr).)This estimate is larger than the AUC because the top of each trapezoid is above the actual curve through the points. A better approximation can be obtained by using more points or by fitting the data with a better function. One such function is a sequence of parabolas (Simpson's rule). Another for these data is the sum of three exponentials (see Table E.9). The "correct" AUC is 4.07 $\mu mol\,hr\,litre^{-1}$. 10-15% accuracy is often adequate.

In this table the areas are calculated directly from the data points. With real, imperfect data it would be better to put a smooth curve through the points and then superimpose the trapezoids onto the smooth curve.

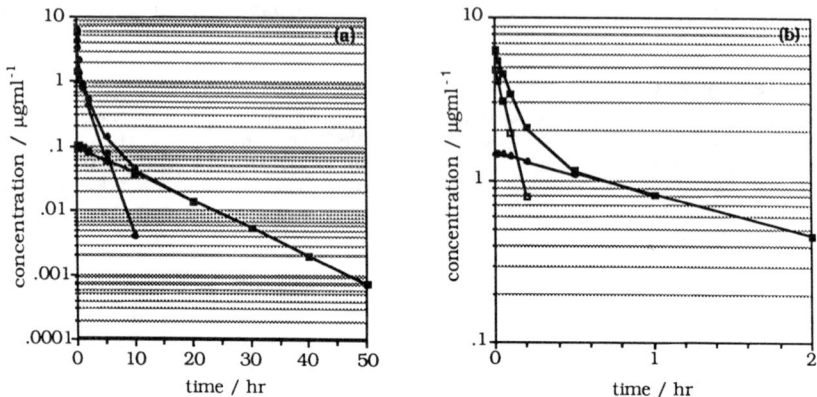

Figure E.3 Plasma concentration versus time following a 10 mg dose of methotrexate. Fitting with a sum of three exponentials. Part (a) shows the data, C, the terminal phase line, C_z and the line corresponding to the intermediate phase. The data with the terminal phase line subtracted, the intermediate phase line, and the initial phase line are shown in part (b). Curve peeling is rarely sufficiently accurate to determine all the constants for three exponentials. It works here because the three rate constants differ from each by at least factors of three and accurate data are available over a 10,000 fold range of concentrations.

$2 \cdot 10^{-8}$ mmol litre^{-1} is

$$t = \frac{1}{\lambda_z} \ln\left(\frac{C_0}{C}\right) = \frac{1}{0.097\,\text{hr}^{-1}} \ln\left(\frac{2.5\,\text{mmol litre}^{-1}}{2 \cdot 10^{-8}\,\text{mmol litre}^{-1}}\right) = 121\,\text{hr}$$

A dose sufficient to produce a concentration of 1 mmol litre^{-1} at the end of 6 hr will produce toxic concentrations for 5 days.

(3) High dose methotrexate is administered by intravenous infusion. The infusion rate to maintain 1 mmol litre^{-1} is

$$R_{in} = CL \cdot C_{ss} = 5.4\,\text{litre hr}^{-1} \cdot 10^{-3}\,\text{mol litre}^{-1} = 5.4\,\text{mmol hr}^{-1} = 2.45\,\text{g hr}^{-1}.$$

By 24 hr (18 hr after the end of the infusion) the fall in concentration is in the terminal phase and for t starting at the time of the sample

$$C(t) = C(24\,\text{hr})\,e^{-\lambda_z t}$$

Table E.10 Curve peeling for the plasma concentration vs time data for methotrexate. These data are plotted in Fig. E.3.

Time / hr	Concentration / μmol litre^{-1}				
	C	C_z	C - C_z	C_2	C_1
0.00	-	0.10	-	1.47	4.80
0.02	5.56	0.10	5.46	1.45	4.01
0.05	4.59	0.10	4.49	1.43	3.06
0.10	3.44	0.099	3.34	1.39	1.95
0.20	2.20	0.098	2.10	1.31	0.79
0.50	1.24	0.095	1.15	1.10	
1.00	0.91	0.091	0.82	0.82	
2.00	0.54	0.082	0.45	0.45	
5.00	0.14	0.062	0.08	0.08	
10.00	0.042	0.038			
20.00	0.014	0.0143			
30.00	0.0054	0.0054			
40.00	0.0020	0.0020			
50.00	0.0007	0.0007			

The three rate constants are $\lambda_1 = 9.00$ hr^{-1}, $\lambda_2 = 0.59$ hr^{-1}, and $\lambda_z = 0.097$ hr^{-1}.

or

$$t = \frac{1}{\lambda_z} \ln\left(\frac{C(24\,hr)}{C(t)}\right) = \frac{1}{0.097}\ln\left(\frac{2 \cdot 10^{-5}\,mol\,litre^{-1}}{2 \cdot 10^{-8}}\right) = 71\,hr.$$

The increase in concentration during the infusion can be described approximately using a beaker model

$$C = C_{ss}\,(1 - e^{-\lambda_z t}) = 1\,mmol\,litre^{-1}\,(1 - 0.56) = 0.44\,mmol\,litre^{-1}.$$

A more accurate value can be obtain using the equations from Section S4.3 and the values for the intercepts and rate constants for the three exponentials. The values of C_1/D, C_2/D, and C_z/D, are 0.22 litre^{-1}, 0.067 litre^{-1}, and 0.0045 litre^{-1} respectively. Thus

$$C = 5.4\,mmol\,hr^{-1}\left(\frac{1}{5.4\,litre\,hr^{-1}} - 0.22\,litre^{-1}\frac{0}{9\,hr^{-1}} - \right.$$

$$\left. 0.067\,litre^{-1}\frac{0.029}{0.059\,hr^{-1}} - 0.0045\,litre^{-1}\frac{0.56}{0.097\,hr^{-1}}\right)$$

$$C = 0.68\,mmol\,litre^{-1}.$$

E.3.11   Doxorubicin

The Fibonacci series is set out in the second column of Table E.11. The dose reaches the MTD = $5 \cdot LD_{10} = 50 \cdot$ (entry level) on the 11th step. Using the entry level dose, LD_{10}, as the test dose the predicted MTD is $(10)(5)/0.8 = 62.5$ times larger. Thus the first step of escalation in the geometric series method would increase the dose by a factor of $\sqrt{62.5} \approx 8$. For the extended factors of two series (repeated 100% increases) 40% of the predicted MTD is 25 times the entry level. This would be exceeded after 5 steps, so the next would be a 50% increase. The series are continued in the Table.

E.3.12   Carboplatin

(1) The clearance for free platinum can be calculated from the free concentrations as dose/(area under the curve) = 10.2 litre hr^{-1} = 170 ml min^{-1}. The renal clearance is 65% of this value, i.e. 110 ml min^{-1} which is slightly less than normal GFR. The terminal phase half-life is 3.3 hr. The terminal phase volume of distribution is about $CL \cdot t_{1/2,z}/0.69 =$ 170 ml min$^{-1} \cdot 3.3$ hr/0.69 = 49 litre. As this value is substantially larger than plasma volume and the terminal phase is reached quickly, it is apparent that carboplatin can enter and leave tissues rapidly. However, these data do not specify the rate at which it can enter cells.

(2) Initially all of the platinum in plasma is free and because most is excreted as carboplatin, free platinum in plasma is intact drug. After 24 hr when 65% has been excreted the total platinum concentration in plasma is 2 μmol litre^{-1} and almost all of this platinum cannot pass through an ultrafiltration membrane, i.e. it is bound to the plasma proteins. This

Table E.11 Dose escalation series for doxorubicin.The initial dose (in mg m$^{2)}$ equals one tenth the mouse LD_{10}

| Step Number | modified Fibonacci | | geometric mean | extended factors of 2 |
	step factor	$\frac{D}{D_{initial}}$	$\frac{D}{D_{initial}}$	$\frac{D}{D_{initial}}$
1	2	2	8	2
2	1.67	3.34	16	4
3	1.5	5.01	24	8
4	1.4	7.01	34	16
5	1.33	9.33	45	32
6	1.33	12.4	59	48
7	1.33	16.5		
8	1.33	21.9		
9	1.33	29.2		
10	1.33	38.9		
11	1.33	51.6		

binding differs from that normally seen with drugs because it is effectively irreversible. As the volume of distribution for the plasma proteins is 8 to 9 litre, the amount of carboplatin present bound to plasma proteins is likely to be near $2\,\mu mol\,litre^{-1} \cdot 8\,litre = 16\,\mu mol$. Roughly 35% of the dose is still in the body at this time thus the fraction of the drug remaining that is bound to the plasma proteins is approximately $16\,\mu mol/(0.35 \cdot 1.87\,mmol) = 0.025$. The rest is sequestered inside cells or bound to macromolecular components of the tissues. Carboplatin is eliminated from plasma primarily by renal excretion, but also partly by sequestration or effectively irreversible binding.

(3) When renal function is impaired the clearance will be decreased and the area under the curve increased. The obvious suggestion for a dose adjustment procedure is to keep dose/CL constant, i.e. to adjust the doses to keep the AUC constant. The rate of renal excretion can be predicted if a method is available to measure GFR. The relation derived taking the non-renal clearance into account is $D = AUC \cdot (GFR + 25)$ for D in mg, AUC in $mg\,min\,ml^{-1}$, and GFR in $ml\,min^{-1}$.

INDEX